DEDICATION

To the near-century old people who remember what history books do not contain.

To family members who take time to discover delightful stories and secrets to living from their elders.

To the memory of each who have lived life to its fullest.

To friend and family who show us how to live our dying.

To tireless caregivers and those who choose service to the elderly as their life work.

To the host of compassionate volunteers who use time, talents, and skills to minister to elder persons in their midst.

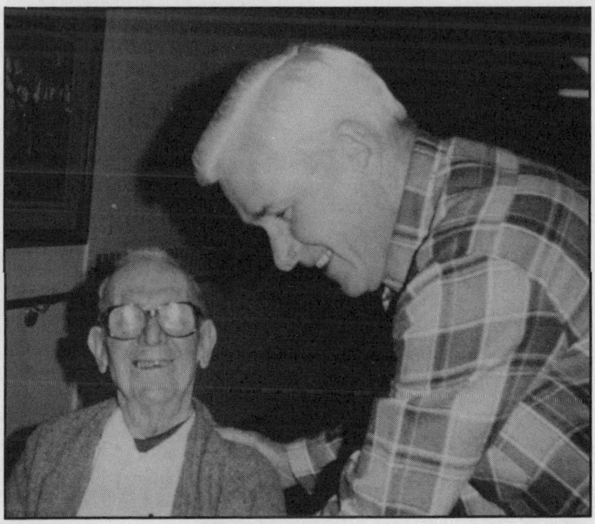

CALL MY NAME . . . TAKE MY HAND

Recipes for Caregivers

A Manual of "how-to", "what-to-do", "where-to-find"
helps for caregiving

Laura R. Hess

"wingborne"

diaconal productions

York, Pennsylvania

1991

Call My Name . . . Take My Hand

Other "wingborne" diaconal productions:

Linking Links: Persons Who Prepare Others for Caregiving

20+ Instant Lesson Plans
© 1992

The Linker, A Handbook for the Administrator/Director of an Intergenerational Training Event

"Link" the Generations with Love +

© 1993

Second Printing

ISBN # 0-9629755-2-4

FOREWORD

Annette Logan **David L. Reed**

Recreation is essential for human beings. Recreation should be fun, a way of keeping in touch with others, and with oneself. For those who are cut off from their accustomed life and ways of spending their days, it is more than essential. It is like air and water; there is no life without it.

Because the creation of fun is not as simple as it would seem to be, because the care of others is time-and-energy consuming just in the meeting of basic needs, this book has been written. Recreation demands imagination, ingenuity, and creativity. We are all in short supply of these occasionally. This book can stimulate ideas for activities for home caretakers who have never had to do this, as well as, put professional recreation therapists in touch with the fun of recreation. Even the most creative people need "cookbooks" of activities to help when we have "programmers' block".

Everyone who needs care is cut off from the main stream of life. This isolation may last only a few days or a lifetime. Recreation can relieve the tedium of empty hours, connect the person with the outside world and with other people, provide an increase in self esteem, teach new skills, and provide an outlet for physical and mental abilities. It can alleviate frustration and tension. Yes, it is certainly therapy, but it is much more than just meeting goals and objectives.

This book will help caregivers, recreation therapists, family, and friends to meet those needs for people who find it difficult, if not impossible, to meet them for themselves. It is full of ideas and information presented in an easy format.

Annette Logan, Ed.D.,
Recreation and Leisure
Associate Professor
York College of Pennsylvania

FOREWORD (Cont'd)

Each person has the right to really live, not just exist.

We all need to love and be loved, unconditionally. Sometimes we are on the giving end and sometimes we are on the receiving end.

Needs are different. Personalities are different. Abilities are different. In all of life we must remember that life is a gift from God, and "But for the grace of God there go I."

In gratefulness for our blessings, we should have compassion for those whose lives we touch.

Both the receiver and the giver of care needs love and understanding. An empty pitcher needs to be filled to provide water to quench thirst. It isn't enough to minister without feeling. We must care and give our services with love, with compassion and with joy.

This book provides many recipes to feed the body, mind and soul.

Adapt ideas from this book, minister with your whole being and discover that "It is more blessed to give than receive."

David L. Reed, N.H.A.
Executive Director
United Methodist
Continuing Care Services
Lewisburg, PA

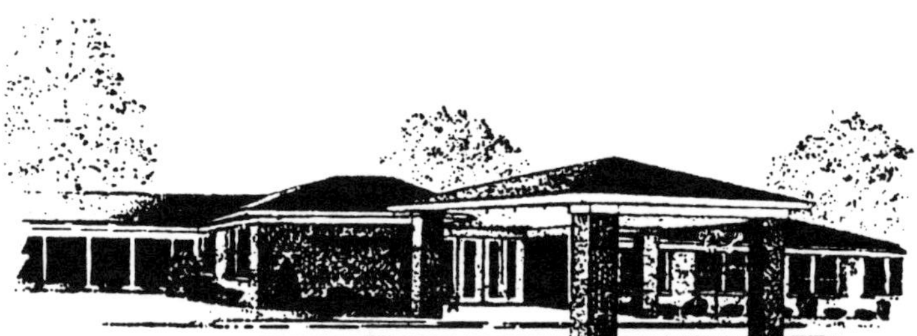

PREFACE

Recently, while visiting a guest in a nursing home, I noted a new resident in that room. I was about to leave, but seemed drawn to the far bedside. To my surprise it was Marie who returned to the home for a second time. "Marie Keller!" I said, as if greeting a long-lost friend. I took her hand in mine. A tear trickled down her cheek. "I can no longer sit up" she said. "I have osteoporosis." I shall miss the good times we shared on Friday evenings.

Some weeks later her picture appeared in the morning paper along with an article regarding letter writing to troops in Saudi Arabia. Still bed-fast, one would quickly recognize her smile. She had just received a letter from the soldier to whom she had written. Several letters were exchanged. She still enjoyed friends for they would come to her room for Bible study led by the chaplain. Marie's inner spirit continued to be vibrant to her last day. I never pass an open doorway without remembering the time I clasped her hand and called her name, for inside each open door their dwells one for whom these simple gestures — a name and a hand — can bring assurance: "I am not forgotten."

PERSONAL WORDS TO THE PRIMARY CAREGIVER

Ann, Charles, Virginia, Ralph, James, Leslie, Jean . . .

You provide care in your home for an aged, or disabled family member, or friend. You perform many tasks such as, bathing, dressing, cooking, cleaning and laundry. You handle finances, give shots, take blood pressure, give medications, change dressings. You run errands, shop and are the source of information to family members and friends near and far. You have little time left over for play.

Why do you do it? Because of your love for that person and the contentment he or she finds in familiar surroundings. Or because of the high cost of outside care. And it is rewarding, though stressful.

As primary caregiver, you need assistance from family, friends, community, or church. You and your loved one will benefit if you take advantage of help that may be available to you. You are not a failure if your loved one ultimately needs placement in a nursing home.

Locate aides to assist you. There are teens out there on whom you might call. You will be doing them a favor. Education systems are encouraging them to volunteer, to raise money for charity. Many teens have been trained in home nursing, candy-striping, CPR and first aid. They learn that money is not the first priority to happiness but giving of themselves can be. With guidance they will serve you well.

Helps in this book can be shared with each who will assist you as well as provide you with "recipes" to enrich and enliven the days of those for whom you care.

A WORD TO THOSE WHO PROFESSIONALLY SERVE AGING INDIVIDUALS

You and the institution where you are at work should be lauded when you plan for the social, recreational and mental stimulation for each guest. Keep seeking adequate budget for the kinds and numbers of activities you need to meet the diversity of the residents under your care. Encourage community organizations, teens, even children, to volunteer their help. Do you remember learning somewhere along the way that there are four basic human needs: security, response, recognition and adventure? And that every individual needs at one time to belong and another time to be separate?

I offer this book to serve your needs, and to facilitate the enjoyment and fullness of life of countless persons who deserve to live fully and contentedly all of the days of their lives.

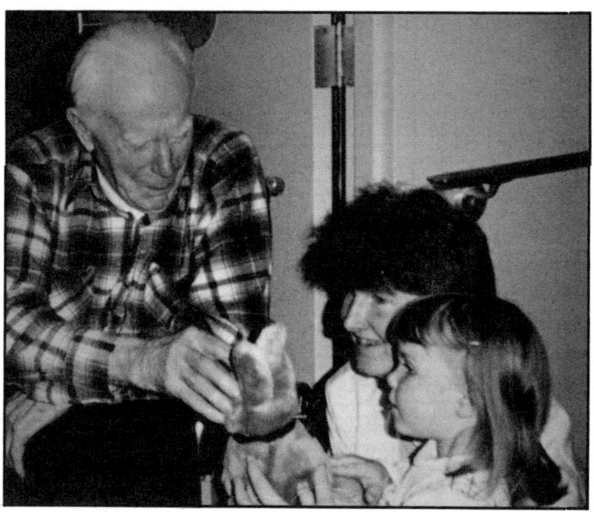

TABLE OF CONTENTS

Foreword

Preface

Table of Contents

Introduction

PART I.

ORIENTATION

SERVE THOSE WHO LOSE TOUCH 11

Develop Reality Orientation Skills 12

Understand and Serve Alzheimer's Patients 16

COMMUNICATE WITH HEARING-IMPAIRED AND DEAF PERSONS 19

Understand Hearing Loss 19

Plan for Hard-of-Hearing and Deaf Persons 20

MOTIVATE TO MEET PSYCHOSOCIAL NEEDS 23

Program for Remotivation 24

CARE FOR THE TERMINALLY ILL 26

Explore Hospice 26

PART II.

ACTIVITIES FROM 'A' to 'Z'

A —ADDRESS, AGE, ANTICIPATION, AUCTION, AUTOMOBILES 30

B —BEES, BIRDS, BOOKS 33

C — CHILDREN, CRAFTS, CURRENT EVENTS 36
D — DANCE, DEATH, DOLLS 39
E — EDUCATION, ENERGIZERS, EVENING, EXERCISES . . . 42
F — FAMILY TABLE, FAVORITE THINGS, FLOWERS, FINGERSPELLING 44
G — GAMES, GARDENING, GROUPINGS 47
H — HISTORY, HOUSE AND HOME, HUMOR 50
I — INTERGENERATIONS, INVENTIONS, INVITATIONS . . . 52
J — JAM AND JELLY, JIGSAW PUZZLES 54
K — KITCHENS, KINFOLK, KNITTING 56
L — LEARNING, LETTER-WRITING, LISTENING 58
M — MEALTIMES, MOUNTAINS, MUSIC 60
N — NAME ORIGINS, NEWSPAPERS 63
O — OCCUPATIONS 66
P — PARTIES, PETS, POETRY 68
Q — QUILTS, QUILTING 73
R — READING, RECORD-KEEPING, RELIGION 74
S — SEASONS, SENSES, STORYTELLING 76
T — TASTING, TOURING 79
U — USEFUL INFORMATION 80
V — VALIDATION, VACATIONS, VISITORS, VOLUNTEERS . 84
W — WAITING, WONDERING, WORSHIPPING 86
X — XMAS PROGRAMMING 88
Y — YOU, YOURSELF 89
Z — ZEBRAS, ZOOS, ZODIAC 90
Acknowledgements
Appendix

INTRODUCTION

Why this manual for caregivers? From earlier experiences and recent conversations with persons at work in old or new health-care facilities or long-term care centers comes a constant lament: "We soon exhaust our resources. We need ideas for content. We need additional aides, volunteers. We need a simple means of orienting these volunteers, as well as new workers."

The expressed need comes at crucial time throughout society. It is a time when the NOW generation (those accustomed to immediate gratification) become caretakers and givers. This ME generation born in the sixties had little time to explore values of previous generations. They grew up in the age of the technological explosion. This need comes with the birth of a new age — persons living ninety and one hundred plus years. But more importantly, it comes before millions of people leave us who knew the world before advancements in mechanization and technology and the advent of television. This older generation has secrets for living and rich life-experiences that today's generations might find significant. The intent of this book is to inspire persons to serve the long-lived, and experience the satisfaction and reward that will come as they serve.

Thus, *Recipes for Caregivers* becomes a handy resource for those wanting to enrich persons' latter years. It is compiled and written during a period of first-hand experience as an activity aide in a health-care facility where caregivers foster holistic health for the residents.

Activities/recreation are prescribed as necessary by state inspection and review boards toward meeting psychosocial needs of those living in a long-time health-care facility. They are no longer an unnecessary or least costly item in a home for care of the elderly. Opportunities for recreation and social activities affect the continued well-being of all persons at any age or stage of life whether healthy or not.

The book contains two parts:

Part I is an orientation for the caregiver, new to the limitations of many members of the aging population. It deals with the following types of limitations prevalent among aging persons for a variety of reasons: namely, persons who lose touch with past and present realities, or cannot deal with usual daily living because of Alzheimer's disease;

persons with communication problems, hearing impairment the most prevalent; those experiencing boredom, lethargy, and lack of motivation. Finally, the needs of terminally ill persons, when physical ministrations cease.

Part II describes a hundred activities, — "recipes" from A to Z. Two or three activities fall under each letter of the alphabet. Some activities are idea starters and suggestions. Others describe the actual happening. There are many with "how-to" directions. You will meet motivated people involved in activity. Note the nuances of caring in settings that ennoble and enrich, even as they help to heal.

This book provides a wealth of resources for use in any setting: private home, day-care center, group home, retirement village, assistive-living facility, nursing or rehabilitation center.

The caregivers are family members of all ages: children, youth, adults, friends, visitors, volunteers, nurses aides, housekeepers, food providers, recreation therapists, activity-department staff, home health-care nurses, hospice volunteers and clergypersons.

These helps are presented to benefit persons who have recouperative needs, — those who use wheelchairs, wear glasses, have hearing aids, endure long, lonely hours, experience a little confusion and find much need for a warm hand, a caring heart and listening ears.

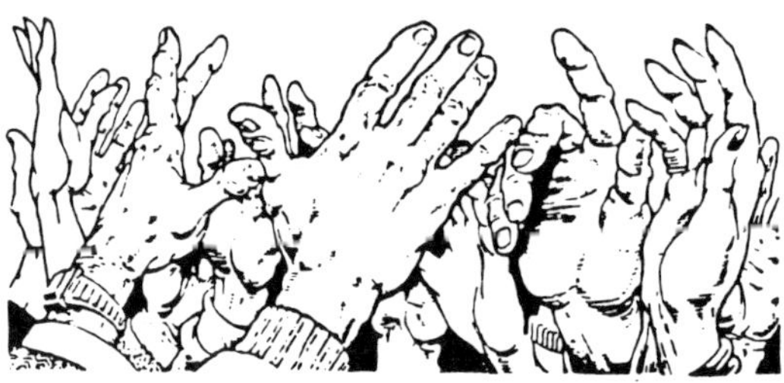

PART I

ORIENTATION

SERVE THOSE WHO LOSE TOUCH

GENERAL REALITY ORIENTATION

ALZHEIMER PATIENT'S

COMMUNICATE WITH HEARING-IMPAIRED PERSONS

UNDERSTAND HEARING LOSS

PLAN FOR HARD-OF-HEARING AND DEAF PERSONS

MOTIVATE TO MEET PSYCHOSOCIAL NEEDS

PROGRAM FOR REMOTIVATION

CARE FOR THE TERMINALLY ILL

EXPLORE HOSPICE

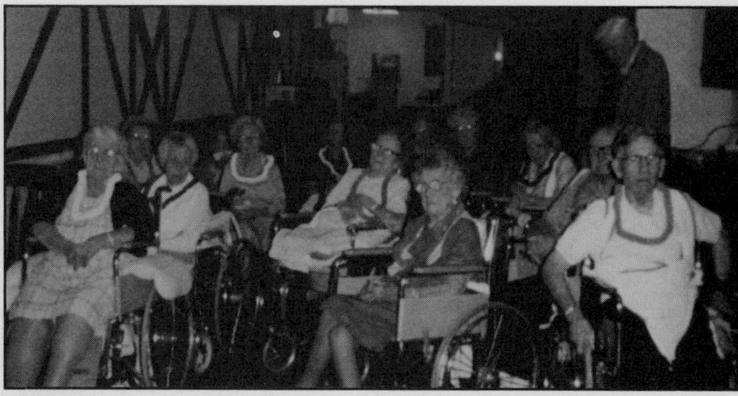

SERVE THOSE WHO LOSE TOUCH

Persons of Western culture are habit-oriented, time-and-schedule directed, often to a point that the clock and calendar guide and control them. Travelers look at an itinerary and comment, as does the movie, *Around the World in 80 Days,* and "if it's Belgium, it must be Tuesday."

We all need to know who we are, where we are, and what time it is. Remember a morning when the alarm did not go off? Or you had no watch and had no idea what time it was? Not knowing the time of day, the day of the week, where you were taken after an accident et cetera contribute to confusion for the most alert individual. The people for whom reality orientation is most appropriate are those who are confused or disoriented for many reasons — stroke, injury, brain syndrome, sensory deprivations, or organic-cerebral deficiency resulting from arteriosclerosis or over-medication.

A reality orientation program, often referred to as R.O., helps deal with problems that result from loss, grief, boredom, fear, and lack of motivation.

Being confused, isolated, withdrawn can be temporary. Confused individuals can improve. Unfortunately, a number of people suffer unnecessarily from treatable and reversible states of confusion.

For example: An elderly gentleman meets with an accident in a strange city while visiting his son. Setting his broken hip necessitates heavy sedation. He awakens in a hospital room disoriented and confused. Unless a knowledgeable doctor stops sedation (tranquilizers) that are routinely given and explains to the patient where he is, addresses him by name, and outlines what has happened to him, the old man is likely to be labeled *senile* and given even more drugs, aggregating his confusion and agitation.

Or a principal of an elementary school in her sixties slows down physically and mentally, slips into a confused state, and neglects her personal hygiene. Diagnosed as senile, she can be saved from a nursing home only by an expert who recognizes the condition as depression and effectively treats it. Depression or acute emotional stress such as that following the loss of a loved one is very common among older adults and often goes unrecognized and untreated.

DEVELOP REALITY ORIENTATION SKILLS

Repetition and consistency are musts when an individual needs help in bringing reality out of confusion. Repeat again and again facts we usually take for granted. Expect appropriate behavior and response. Inform as to what, where, how, and when. Talk to and not at the individual. Watch for results from administering regular reality orientation techniques. Is the individual showing increased awareness of him-or-herself and of his/her surroundings? Is the individual showing increased interest in his/her own affairs?

Every one who comes in contact with that person is an important member of his/her growing well-being. This includes families of patients, medical and nursing personnel, dietitians, volunteers, maintenance workers, housekeepers, pastors, et cetera.

REALITY ORIENTATION SKILLS NEEDED AT HOME — TWENTY-FOUR HOURS A DAY.

Remind the confused individual throughout the day of his name, your name, the date, his location (address) what the next meal is, e.g., "Good morning, Grandmother. We will be having breakfast soon. It is 8:00 A.M. We will eat breakfast at 8:30."

Involve all family members, even young children, in correcting the disoriented person in a respectful manner. Prepare friends and neighbors to use basic principles — Introduce self and correct misunderstandings. Example: to Grandfather, "I'm not Johnny, I'm Philip."

Acquire the habit of announcing events: "It's time for your bath, John," and give all directions: "The bathroom is this way. I'll push your wheelchair to the bathroom, John."

Correct patient's disoriented remarks immediately. "I'm your daughter Ruth, not your mother. Do I remind you of her?"

Keep changes to a minimum. Avoid moving furniture around.

Spend ten-to-twenty minutes a day in a discussion with the disoriented person. Talk about place, and time, and have a chart with day of week, next meal and next holiday visible. Place calendar, magazines and family pictures within sight and touch.

REALITY ORIENTATION DISCUSSION TOPICS

Whether in one's own home, or in a nursing facility, physicians may indicate the patient's need for reality orientation. In one's own home, any family member, visitor or friend may engage the elderly person in conversation that serves to orientate the individual to realities — past, and present. The list of topics below serves as a starter for conversations.

You may add other topics to develop into five- or ten-minute conversations, supplementing conversations with old photos, news clippings, or other tangible objects adds curiosity and interest.

Name — Who gave you your name? For whom are you named?

Address — present, past, other places you remember living?

Time — season, month, day, year. Calendars, favorite days.

Birthdates — When? Where? How old? A favorite birthday.
Who remembered? How?

Mealtimes — What is your favorite meal? Favorite foods?
What was your latest meal? What did you eat?
Compare eating at home with dining out.
What are your favorite restaurants?

Your home — Describe a house you have lived in. A favorite room.

School Days — First day of school, teachers, building.

Work — What kind of work did you do?
What work do your sons, daughters, grandchildren do now.
What kind of employment did your parents have?

Pay Check — How much was your first one?
How much would it be today?
How did you spend it?

Responsibilities — What were yours as a child? A youth?
As a parent? A homeowner? Husband? Wife?
Do you have responsibility today? What?
Who assists you?

Church — Recall experiences of baptism, confirmation, marriage, divorce, death, funerals.

Feelings — Discuss happy and sad feelings, et cetera.

Weather — Talk about changes, storms, rainbows.

In some nursing facilities groups of patients (five or six) are brought together for a half hour of reality orientation a day. In another facility reality-orientation tapes are made and taken to individuals, thus increasing the opportunities for reality orientation. Tapes may be used where three or four come together in a common meeting place, requiring minimal preparation ahead of time and can be directed by a volunteer.

MEET SOME NURSING HOME RESIDENTS

The following residents participated daily in a reality orientation class in a nursing home. As you read the descriptions of each, you will no doubt exclaim that you know that individual. She was the image of your grandmother. If you have not met these individuals, you may come to love and care for one just like Edith, or May.

EDITH L.

Many call her Grandma. Her thin white hair pulled to the top of her head rests in a small, tight knot. Her glasses slide down her nose causing her to look out on her world over top of them. Her frail body is agile enough to pitter-patter through her room, to and from her roommate's corner and then to the doorway to watch for the arrival of the meal-delivery cart.

When in a reality orientation group Edith puts her head down on the table and sighs, "Oh, dear!" or responds, "I'm just a mess." Another persistent lament — failing eyesight. Her self-preoccupation blocks out what is going on around her. She often causes her peers to feel she does not like to be with them.

A break-through to understanding comes in an reality-orientation session when she sits straight up on her chair, exclaiming in no uncertain words, "You are all making a monkey out of me by asking again and again where I live. What day is it? What is my next meal?" "You know, I feel like a monkey, too" responds the leader. With that Edith's expression changes to a broad grin. Eyes twinkling, she throws back her head in a roar of laughter.

Another time, while listening to a beautifully poignant story about training guide dogs for the blind, Edith's head goes into her hands and back down on the table as if in pain. All eyes focus on her. The story aside — the conversation turns to feelings and fears persons have of the unknown, of blindness, death . . .

The subject of grandchildren usually one prompting stories recalled from the past is not so for Edith. She tells of the tragedies in her life — the loss of two husbands, one a merciless death while driving a cab. In the early years of marriage, her loss of babies. She had no grandchildren.

Somehow, we know why she deserves the endearing term of "Grandma" from each of her caregivers. Over her spectacles and from a dejected countenance, there comes a broad, mischievous smile; a hand reaches for the face of the one before her, pulling it down to implant a warm kiss. She is indeed a grandmother to many who give her care.

MAY O.

One is immediately captivated by her face
Such myriad lines etched deeply and beautifully thereon
  can scarcely be matched.
A face of quiet dignity upon first glance,
But more to come in time.
A woman of word is she.
Not only of word but of deep and gentle humor.
Eyes dance with mischief and jollity.
Both lucid and reflective moments are so short
  that they often pass unobserved.
O, how in love with life is she
And how intensely stubborn at times.
Sage, yet often unrelated are her utterings —
That her parents believed in good education
A fact repeated ten times over,
Soon falls on deaf ears.
Rhythm fills her frail body when music begins.
To dance and dance — eyes twinkle with memories.
She reflects the words shown in her eyes:
"How my father liked to dance, and so did we!"

Five minutes her interest span.
"I must be going. I'm expecting company."
Rising from her chair, regally poised with cane in hand
To her room she returns.

UNDERSTAND AND SERVE ALZHEIMER PATIENTS

They enjoyed so many things together. Husband and wife things, and they had many friends. They were always together in worship on a Sunday morning. Then she was no longer there. Upon inquiry you learn of a new affliction which renders the afflicted one totally helpless to direct affairs, or manage dressing to meet the day. The disease is known as Alzheimers.

Ruth, when in her late fifties sent to all her friends a copy of a Christmas greeting she had designed many years ago. Little did the recipients who lived far away realize it would be the last touch with the old Ruth who taught school, participated actively in church and community, married, reared a beautiful family. Last summer she came with her husband to visit the home of her earlier years. Those who came to see her were distressed to discover total personality obliteration. While totally dependent on her husband for everything she maintains her sweet disposition and smile.

Alzheimer's Disease

Until quite recently one of the most common and generally pervasive maladies of aging was termed *senility*. Today, this condition is spoken of as Alzheimer's Disease. Over one half of the individuals in nursing homes is afflicted.

This intellectual impairment affects ability to learn, remember, understand, reason, imagine, think abstractly, make judgments, and draw conclusions from, or about, the environment.

Early symptoms are increased difficulty in doing simple tasks, and forgetfulness, e.g., "Where did I park my car?" Others are increased agitation, mood changes, and restlessness, even an inability to care for oneself. At this point the stress brought to bear on family members increases. It is important that caregivers have breaks from the daily care. Psychologists suggest special attention be given to their survival needs.

To know an indivisual who loses total touch with the past, cannot retain the present and has no future, prompts search and research for help in care and curbing the development of Alzheimer's disease.

About the Person Afflicted

This individual can no longer meet needs of spouse or children. No two individuals are affected at the same rate. Each needs to continue in an orderly daily routine, in an environmentally controlled facility. He/she requires a balance of nourishment, fluids and exercise. After the age of forty or forty-five, recollection of small details may decline even though more permanent memories remain vividly intact.

Suggestions to family members upon first signs of memory failure:

Help eliminate distractions. Give simple responses such as "Come back at four o'clock."

Plan for activity. Inactivity breeds depression and one day blends into another. Assist the family member in writing a diary, adding something new each day. Date each entry, or write a news event every day.

Play association games together. The author recalls a hospital experience some years ago. Her nurse's name was Miss Drake. She was proud to introduce the nurse to her family the next day. "Meet Miss Crane" she said. The nurse laughed. "Drake is my name. Both are names of long-legged birds and I resemble both of them." All laughed and the ice was broken.

Encourage good organization. Whether disorganization is a cause or result of memory loss, it is essential to develop systematic ways of remembering appointments; where one placed things; times for paying bills, and make a list of things to do each day.

Prepare ahead. Before going to a meeting, entertaining guests, visiting grandchildren, review the names of who will be there.

Help the person to remember, e.g., "Mother, today is the day for your doctor's appointment. We'll leave the house at 10:30 A.M. Your appointment is at 11:00 A.M."

Where memory loss is evident, look for possible physical causes. Medicine for certain illnesses may seriously affect memory.

Long-term care and the Alzheimer's patient.

A spouse or family member is hard-pressed to locate a long-term-care facility adequate to meet needs of the Alzheimer's patient. Because this person wanders away and can become lost, close supervision and containment within a safe area is necessary. One health-care corporation seeks to provide special units for residents afflicted with this disease, naming them Arcadia I and II. These units with wide halls display each individual's picture at eye-level under the room number at the side of the door. Controlled atmosphere, soft lighting and quiet music fill the enclosed areas of the Arcadia units. Individuals are free to roam in and out of doors to a patio and garden area that are within safe bounds. In these units, staff members provide twelve hours of activity a day, literally living with the more mobile individuals. As more physical deteriation sets in persons are moved to Arcadia II, where they may be confined to a wheelchair, but still have freedom of mobility and scheduled activity. Most centers prepared to care for Alzheimer patients will provide a family-support program.

The number of services for the Alzheimer's patient and his or her caretaker is increasing. Watch for day-care centers for the afflicted person. Note announcement of a support group for spouses and other family members.

"As a white candle
In a holy place,
So is the beauty
Of an aged face."

COMMUNICATE WITH HEARING-IMPAIRED PERSONS

Ella appears to be the average eighty-year-old widow: white halo, ringed fingers, eyes that follow every move. Soon after she enters a nursing home for physical therapy she can become characterized as stubborn, uncooperative with tendancy for sullenness. Staff looks at her records. *Deaf mute*. She is deaf but *not* mute. One seeking to communicate with her may hear a jumble of sounds and upon closer listening will catch words she is trying to frame in the context of what she perceives.

Ella, is but one of one million, eight hundred thousand plus individuals across the land who is *prelingually* deaf who may eventually need care in a hospital or home. These persons became deaf before learning to talk. They have never heard sounds and words an average child would pick up from the environment. Deafness was a result of high fever, or perchance a mother's exposure to rubella during the first trimester of pregnancy. There are other causes.

Everyone who enters a health-care facility must be informed of resident's rights. Ella would need someone to sign these to her, for her mode of communication is ASL (American Sign Language). Reading level is low, and vocabulary simple. Deaf persons rely on information they can see. Communication, to be effective, must be visible.

UNDERSTAND HEARING LOSS

Hearing loss is the most prevalent, yet least recognized physical ailment that affects people of all ages. It is a hidden handicap. More people have hearing disorders than heart disease, cancer, blindness, kidney disease, tuberculosis, and multiple sclerosis combined. While hearing loss can occur at any age, it is most common in older people and a matter of great concern to those affected.

The Effect of Hearing Loss on the Individual

The person with hearing loss has a problem communicating in groups. That individual experiences discomfort in noisy environments if he or she wears a hearing aid. Most persons have difficulty on the telephone unless phone and aid are properly equipped to accomodate a special problem.

The person experiencing hearing loss has increased physical tension due to sustained hyper-alertness, and increased mental tension aggravated by frequent ringing in the ears.

One's self-confidence is lessened due to inability to accurately perceive information from the environment.

Frequent social withdrawal leads to isolation, anxiety and depression. Denial of a loss or avoidance of that reality frequently heightens the negative effects.

The individual who moves into a new environment such as a hospital or nursing home and does not hear nor understand the caretaker, who in turn does not understand deafness, can become disoriented, frustrated, and have temper tantrums. Such an experience can deter recovery, adjustment to new living situations and contribute to depression and decline.

Effects of Hearing Loss on Others

A communication problem affects both the sender and receiver. Family members living with a hearing-impaired person experience more physical and mental tension as well as increased negative emotions such as anger, anxiety and depression. "Later, I will explain," becomes a way of preventing a scene.

The caretaker loses patience and deters understanding on the part of the deafening individual.

Friends and coworkers begin to reject one who has difficulty hearing, "We'll not invite him," or "She monopolizes conversation so she knows what is going on." A comfortable climate is thus assured, but unwittingly isolates the deaf friend or coworker.

PLAN FOR HARD-OF-HEARING AND DEAF PERSONS

If you are a caregiver, nurse, family member, visitor or volunteer, check your readiness to serve any hearing-impaired person. Here is a list of things to do.

Keep paper and pen handy.
Turn light off and on for attention.
Keep patient's eyeglasses available.
Don't talk with back to window or lamp.
Face patient directly when you talk.

Don't cover mouth with hands.
Do nothing unexpected from behind the patient.
Allow plenty of time for every communication.
Repeat what you say, rephrasing.
Position patient to see what is going on. Prevent isolation.
Never restrict a deaf person's hands.
Give emotional support.
Reassure patient before you leave the room.
Keep your communication simple.

The health care facility that can respond in the affirmative to the following questions is ready to serve the person with a hearing problem.

Does patient's record indicate mode of communcation?

Is there a list of available sign-language interpreters?

Do you place over the bed of a deaf person the mode of communication that person uses: e.g. writes, lip reads, fingerspells, mimes, pictures, or sign language only.

Is a telephone device (TDD) for the deaf available for use? Do you provide close-captioned television?

Do you display the international symbol for the hearing-impaired, thus denoting your readiness to serve the deaf resident or patient?

Secure communication aids

Acquire a hearing aid equipped with a telephone (T) switch, that enhances talking on phone or hearing in a room where there is an audio-loop system.

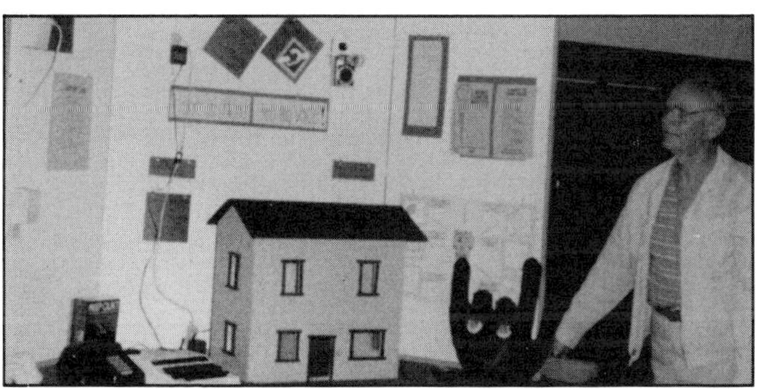

Get an amplifier for use with the telephone. Inquire at your local phone office.

There are devices for listening to television and radio. Ask about the infrared small-room transmittors.

Flashing-light signals for doorbell, phone and alarm clock are available through your local electronic stores. Also smoke alarms that flash.

Many churches, concert halls, theaters and smaller meeting rooms found in hospital and nursing homes are putting in assistive-listening systems which take the desired speech signal directly to the individuals ear, thereby eliminating distracting noises.

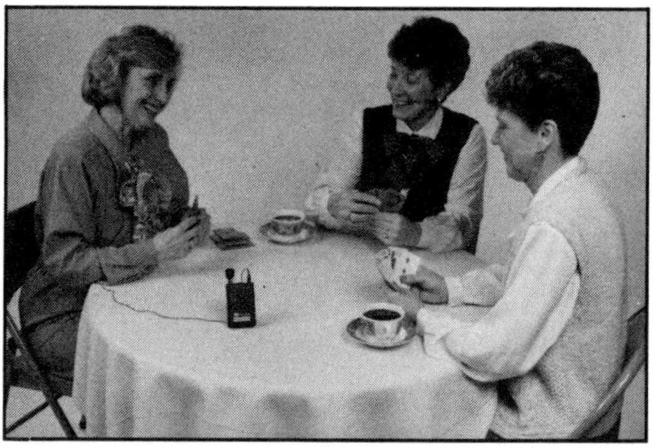

MOTIVATE TO MEET PSYCHOSOCIAL NEEDS

Whether a person lives alone in his or her home, in a personal care facility, or a nursing home, there are times when assistance to a fuller participation in life may be necessary. Even if the individual has a number of disabilities, taking part in social functions planned or spontaneous activities can give him/her a greater sense of well-being. A young-appearing ninety-year-old, who did not believe she should be placed in a nursing home is frequently despondent, but comes alive when its time for an activity to her liking. She regrets that the evening game activity ends all too soon, and often gathers with neighboring residents to visit awhile before retiring. She seeks other ways to keep busy. Remembering volunteer hours with a hospital auxiliary some years ago, she finds her way to the room where the agency newsletter is being prepared for distribution to help and recount previous times of delight in working along side hospital staff in a similar project. After a move to another location in the home, a brief hospital encounter, and resulting disenchantment with living, she died. Discouragement, depression, seeming uselessness, lack of a goal for the day or weeks ahead, feeling unloved, cut-off, abandoned, weariness from body disfunction that may never improve: these are signs that call for remotivation. The caregiver, particularly the primary caregiver, is frequently aware when the cared-for person's motivation is low — all goals reached, a long anticipated event past, not much else to do, no more feeling needed — one's task on earth is finished. The elderly person, living longer than any other person in his family, needs help with new goals and purposes.

Remotivation simply means stimiulating the individual to a heightened degree of interest in what goes on around him.

The caregiver must first respect the right of one to refuse to participate in a remotivating activity and yet needs to administer such treatment advocated by family or physician. To lure, prod, encourage unmotivated individuals to participate in an activity may take skill and patience. To find the key to unlock the closed door to free the listless individual to fuller living is a constant aim of the activity personnel in a home or center caring for aged persons. Physicians may order activities for their patients. Family members request the same.

DEVELOP A PROGRAM WITH MOTIVATIONAL INTENT

Inquire about a remotivation program in a facility where elders reside. Is there a program listed with regularity for persons needing remotivation? Visit to observe a scheduled activity.

Remotivation in a group setting.

Leaders of a remotivation activity are aware of the little ways that encourage and elicit participation. The following are some of them:

Greet each person by name. Give warm welcome. Introduce each one. Invite each person to tell where they used to live. Many persons will take real interest in the new resident. Persons are introduced who do not know each other. Inquire if anyone knows everyone. The leader will introduce himself/herself and tell a sentence or so about himself. Names are important.

Seating for best hearing and visibility is important to insure the participation of each individual. A climate of acceptance of any contribution of any individual during an activity; and assurance and reassurance for the wary person wandering in attention from what is happening in the remotivation session are essentials for a good session.

A stimulating topic, frequently season-related, is presented by the leader. Pictures, slides, simple objects facilitate discussion and recall, and can culminate with each person sharing a story, a memory, or a happening long forgotten. Often a sense of comradary develops as persons share their experiences.

Holidays are times for remotivating individuals. Martha J. watches from her doorway, but refuses to participate in many things going on around her. Halloween would be an exception. She handed packages of popcorn to the steady stream of children who came by in their Halloween costumes, when her residence held a “Safe-Halloween” event for elementary school children. Days and weeks later, she tells everyone she sees about the experience.

There can be long dry spells between special celebrations. Plan for ways to brighten rainy days and long winter hours. Even hold an unbirthday party, or celebrate Christmas in July, inviting grandchildren to sing and bring a package containing a home-made gift.

It’s little things that lift the spirit, nourish and feed the soul and makes the heart sing.

Remotivation in a private home.

The elderly person living with family in his/her own home, needs remotivation. There the family caregivers assume responsibility for motivating activities. They may invite one or two friends to afternoon tea, show a new purchase received by mail-order, do some arm chair shopping, or show recently received pictures of grandchildren. They may fill the house with pleasant aromas; prepare some curiosity-arousing packages; utilize the magic of touching, hugging, tasting, listening; and serve some herbal tea and cookies.

Simple little occurences can eliminate feelings of isolation on the part of the grandparent, while living within the family home. Younger generations can benefit from integrating shared-care into their busy lives.

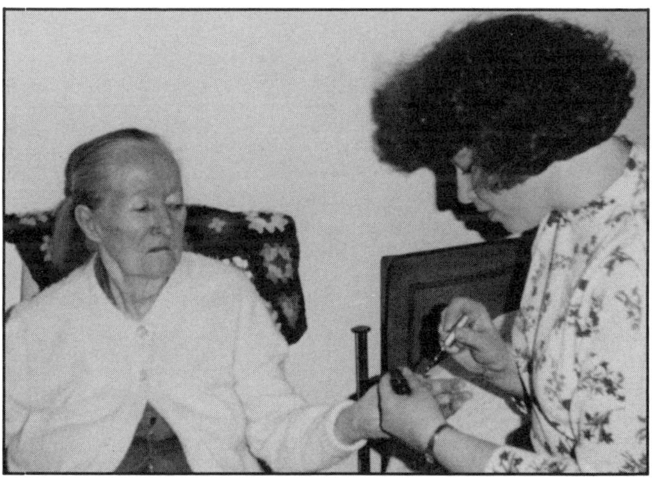

CARE FOR THE TERMINALLY ILL

The journey that begins with the first breath of life is followed with time-filled experiences, to life's last task — that of dying. Most of us recall a first experience with death. A family pet, a classmate, a grandparent. Each personal experience can bring insight, understanding, recollection. Sympathy moves toward empathy, and empathy to caring, and caring to caregiving.

Caregivers from generation to generation have found varied means of rendering support. Many faith communities still sing the Fannie Crosby hymn entitled "Rescue the Perishing." The next phrase in this time-honored poem by the beloved blind poet is "Care for the Dying". One may reflect on what might have been ways of giving care to the individual in his/her latter days in the mid-nineteenth century. In the early 1970's however, a movement began in the United States to meet dying persons needs, improve their quality of life and assure a death with dignity and awareness.

ENTER, HOSPICE

Travelers through the English country-side found places of shelter where they might stop and find rest, and renewal from a long days' journey. These places of shelter for the weary traveler were known by the title: *Hospice*. The term Hospice, borrowed from England, came to describe the program developed within the United States to meet the needs of dying persons.

Death with dignity and a freedom from fear and pain are earmarks of the hospice philosophy. Elements included in Hospice services are pain reduction while maintaining aliveness and alertness, comfort, spiritual ministration, and a holistic approach to patient and family. Local hospitals may offer the services of Hospice to their patient when active treatment ceases. The trained hospice volunteer, assigned to a patient, will then give time and friendship under the direction of a professional team of workers, and will be as near as the telephone to the patient and family members twenty-four hours a day seven days a week; and may be supportive to the family through a period of grieving.

Rules for the Hospice worker.

Allow opportunity to the person to talk.

Don't over-power with your responses and thoughts.

Don't ask. Just do.

Share hurts, fears, concerns.

When solicited share your experience.

Do not dwell on the prognosis.

Encourage and provide for outside interests.

Truly enjoy being with the individual.

Maintain strong, vibrant faith.

Elements in Training

Professional hospice workers are the registered nurse, the home health aide, social worker, physical therapist, occupational therapist, speech therapist and volunteer coordinator. These workers are coordinated by a hospice coordinator. There is a hospice medical director, usually a physician in the community.

These persons make up the Hospice Team responsible for the care of the patient on a daily basis, providing direction to all family members and anyone near to the one to whom the volunteer is giving care.

The hospice volunteer, caregiver, may attend an eleven-week training program set up by the volunteer coordinator. Elements taught in this program include: family dynamics; spiritual/cultural aspects of the community; disease process; grieving process; communication skills; pain. A hands-on experience provides for development of skill in moving, touching, etc. Legal and financial aspects in training including functions of attorney, and tour of funeral home.

The volunteer, aware of self and his/her personal death, is assigned a patient to whom he/she is matched by the professional team who provide coordinated services.

Reflections through the window

For a space of time — two months perhaps, Belle spoke of her lovely new friend. They met following her brief stay at the local hospital. If Belle understood the friend as a "hospice volunteer" it was the friendship that became important. Family lived miles away. The realization that other attacks could send her to the hospital in wee hours of morning, the decision had been made, with here consent, to participate in the Hospice program. The day came when the hospice "friend" moved out of State. Belle's health improved. Now she lives in a personal care home. She still recalls the good times and letters she and "her friend" shared with each other.

Discover Catherine through another window. Catherine died. She did not want to die. There was so much she wanted to do. For a year she experienced rapid decline, calling for friends and family to adjust to changes in physical appearance, even as she made adjustment to diminishing bodily function and ensuing treatments, — always exuding a calm composure to the outside world. In that year she typed newsletters, manuscripts, minutes and planned for the elder programs at her church. She crocheted afghans, embroidered, and produced lavishly. She told the folk at the hospital she did not need a hospice person for there were many who were weekly or daily present to give a hug, squeeze of a hand, share a memory, shop for yarn. Spouse, daughter, pastor would tend her through difficult times. There came a day Catherine said: "I have nothing more to do," seeming to grasp for yet another task. It was the end of that week she died. Christmas came not long after. A traditional Christmas luncheon that might have been in jeopardy became a celebration of her life and presence. Around the fireplace after the meal symbols of life were exchanged. Among them were gifts from Catherine, embroidered with love and care. Most saw her FROM LIFE TO LIFE, and they would be so right.

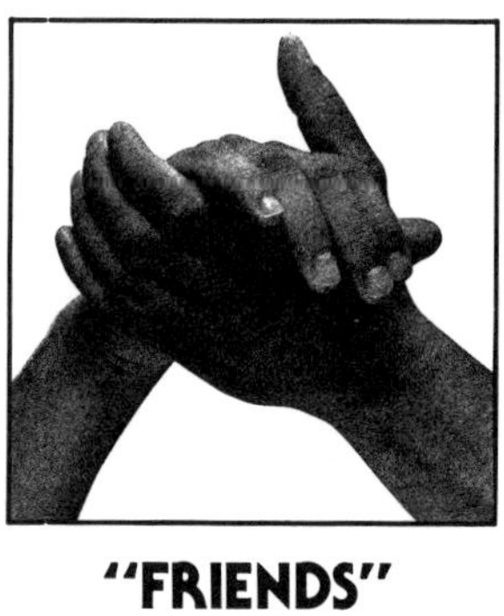

"FRIENDS"

PART II

Read through the activities found in Part II classified according to the alphabet. Make a list of those activities that can motivate the person or persons for whom you share responsibility to give care.

ACTIVITIES FROM A TO Z

INTRODUCTION

A —ADDRESS, AGE, ANTICIPATION, AUCTION, AUTOMOBILES

B —BEES, BIRDS, BOOKS

C —CHILDREN, CRAFTS, CURRENT EVENTS

D —DANCE, DEATH, DOLLS

E —EDUCATION, ENERGIZERS, EVENING, EXERCISES

F —FAMILY TABLE, FAVORITE THINGS, FLOWERS, FINGER-SPELLING

G —GAMES, GARDENING, GROUPINGS

H —HISTORY, HOUSE AND HOME, HUMOR

I —INTERGENERATIONS, INVENTIONS, INVITATIONS

J —JAM AND JELLY, JIGSAW PUZZLES

K —KITCHENS, KINFOLK, KNITTING

L —LEARNING, LETTER-WRITING, LISTENING

M —MEALTIMES, MOUNTAINS, MUSIC

N —NAME ORIGINS, NEWSPAPERS

O —OCCUPATIONS

P —PARTIES, PETS, POETRY

Q —QUILTS, QUILTING

R —READING, RECORD-KEEPING, RELIGION

S —SEASONS, SENSES, STORY-TELLING

T —TASTING, TOURING

U —USEFUL INFORMATION

V —VALIDATION, VACATIONS, VISITORS, VOLUNTEERS

W —WAITING, WONDERING, WORSHIPPING

X —XMAS PROGRAMMING

Y —YOU, YOURSELF

Z —ZEBRAS, ZOOS, ZODIAC

PART II.

IDEAS FROM A TO Z

Activity — whether it be physical, mental, emotional, social, or spiritual — should be recognized as a vital factor in the holistic approach to life and health. Whether one is approaching retirement, living his eighties, recovering from surgery, or is being treated medically or emotionally for chronic complaints, a balance of activity is essential.

Patterns of health care, eventuating to total care in a nursing home from an individual's own home, may not show priority to scheduled activities, nor may some attending physicians. Families whose members have pursued hobbies like reading, playing games, stamp-collecting rate such things as fellowship with others at a game of cards, opportunity to continue knitting, do wood-working, read a good book as essential. Health-producing activities should not be abandoned when physical or mental capacities decline, but should be offered with love, compassion, and skill keeping in mind capabilities of persons. Caregivers experiencing stressful and frustrating periods, need pleasure-producing periods of relief while rendering service to an aging family member, nursing home resident, neighbor or friend.

Many activities from A to Z, listed and followed by simple illustrations, will be familiar. This section is provided to give a useful and handy tool for busy caregivers of their long-lived clientele, family or friends.

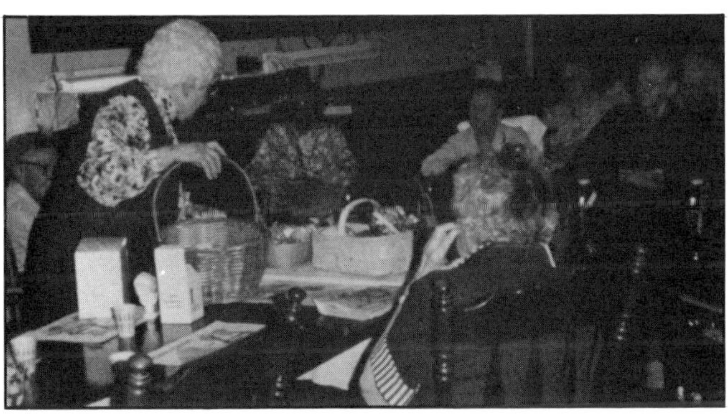

A

ADDRESS
AGE
ANTICIPATION
AUCTION
AUTOMOBILES

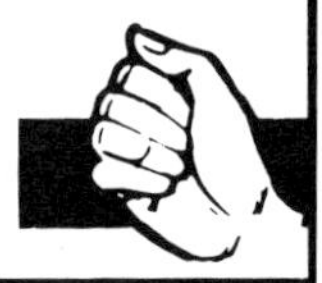

ADDRESS

Persons who have moved from home to nursing home, or even from room to room in a home or nursing home fill with apprehension or anticipation. They may still experience dislocation. It is helpful to talk about addresses — streets, cities, states, even countries — where one has lived, or where one's ancestors lived, and where one's grandchildren are living today. Consider what program you can develop with the theme of addresses.

Play a game. List on chalkboard or newsprint names of states, then cities, then streets, where each person lived. Many will discover "connections" with another: "I didn't know you came here from my home town" or "Do you remember old Sam West, the town barber?" et cetera. Conclude with some references to Thornton Wilder's "Our Town" or listen to a story on tape from Garrison Keillor's book or radio program about Lake Wobegon Days. Locate these in your local library.

AGE

Age is an ever-recurring topic among individuals young and old. Consider a small-group activity built around this theme. Begin with the idea of the Ages of Man. List some of these. Talk about the Prehistoric Age, the Iron Age, the Industrial Age. Many have grown up in the age of agriculture. Many will know the age of technology. Talk about B.C. and A.D., or the age of B.T. or A.T. — before television and after television. Anthropologists rely on carbon dating. What is it?

Pursue another subject: the year you were born. What happened that year? What was it like for your family?

Age is divided into early childhood, later childhood, adolescence, young-middle and older-adults years. Choose an age range and share some stories.

ANTICIPATION

As with children, elders have a penchant for anticipation. In fact, the time of anticipation can be more exciting than the event or happening awaited. Happy hours may be spent planning, talking about, and sharing with others what is going to occur. It is important that the anticipated event is fulfilled.

With older persons the length of time between the planning and the event should be a matter of a few days. When other things intervene, confusion can result. Have a calendar at hand to show date of event. Say, "Today is Wednesday. The party is Saturday. The children are eager to hear some stories about your childhood. Here is paper to write a few notes."

AUCTION

A popular newspaper column is written by an appraiser. Individuals write asking the value of a treasured piece of furniture, china or artifact. The reader is elated to discover the worth of an article that has become a true antique. For many persons whose home is a room, such treasures are but memories. Many still feel the pain of being separated from their homes. Some individuals have chosen what to bring to the personal-care home. Other persons recall a family auction. Talking about it may bring some relief and the ability to accept the present reality.

Invite individuals to a "show and tell" time. Gather a few treasures. Some persons will have an object to bring. Have some pictures of items like a carpet beater, a hand churn, depression glass. Invite a spouse or son or daughter to bring an heirloom. Have a guest appraiser. In conclusion note that age brings increased value. Anna, who often seems embarrassed about her unbelievable age, will find reinforcement and pride as she meets each new day affirming her increased value.

Have an auction of items made by residents. Select an auctioneer from among residents or staff. Allow for much participation and conversation.

AUTOMOBILES

Automobiles have come into existence within the lifetime of most senior citizens. Many will remember the time before the automobile, and their earliest family car. Plan numerous programs using this theme. In a spelling bee spell Cadillac, Porsche, Edsel, Ford, et cetera. The best and worst speller can participate. Gather pictures of automobiles. Pass them around to be identified. Discuss how automobiles changed the life of America. Invite owner of an antique car to speak. Take a bus tour to a museum, or historical society. Have an automobile dealer describe cars of the future. Invite family members to participate with their elderly relative living in a nursing home.

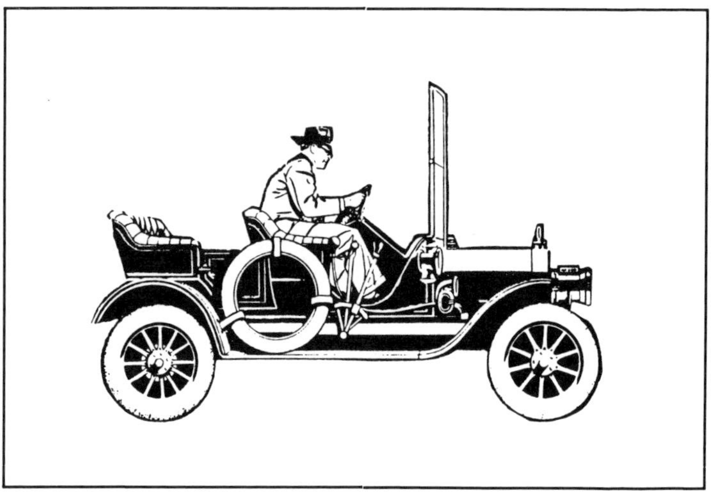

B

BEES
BIRDS
BOOKS

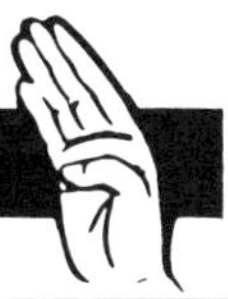

BEES

THE HONEY BEE. The story of the honey bee is a fascinating one. Ask a bee keeper to do a program. There may be a former bee keeper living in your residence. Invite a naturalist from a wild-life preserve to display a sealed-case showing bees at work in a hive. Taste several kinds of honey. Serve herb tea, with honey as sweetner and freshly made biscuits. Listen for honey stories residents relate. Some farm folk may tell of planting buckwheat for honey and for attracting deer that would otherwise destroy a garden.

THE SPELLING BEE. Devise the setting: Sing "School Days", ring an old-fashioned bell, dress the school marm in bonnet and apron pencil behind ear and slate in hand. Begin with song, *"My Country 'tis of Thee."* Salute the flag. Show the award that will go to the best speller. Take pictures.

A spelling bee is a regularly scheduled activity in many health-care facilities. Everyone can spell some words. Place participants in two rows facing each other. For variety, group words by themes, e.g., trees, flowers, birds, et cetera. One row or team will give a word to the persons seated across. That person will spell it. Soon even the persons who declare they cannot spell are involved.

A good speller seldom loses ability to spell. A few moments at the bed-side of an aging former director of nurses, providing a personal spelling bee, gives mental stimulus and relief from boredom.

An intellectually-endowed resident of a health-care center can exhibit unbelievable mood swings from anger and frustration to broad smile and self-satisfaction when engaged in spelling a word or two.

BIRDS

Who has not heralded the robin's song when March breaks winter's hold across the Northland, or a mocking bird outside the window on a summer's night, or the honking of wild geese in Spring or Fall.

The subject of birds can mean many things. Not one bird goes unrecognized by its Maker. Recall the Bible verse: "Look at the birds of the air; they neither sow nor reap nor gather into barns, yet your heavenly Father feeds them. Are you not of more value than they?" (Matthew 6:26). Remember the song, "His Eye is on the Sparrow"?

Plan a program about feathered friends. Invite interested individuals to assist. Someone may belong to the Audubon Society. Find a former bird watcher.

Plans might include a visit to a bird sanctuary or slides of birds and a game to identify them. Keep abreast of what is happening to preserve species — the Bald eagle, for instance.

Obtain recording on tape of bird songs to use at a patient's bedside.

Locate poetry about birds. Some individuals will remember the quatrain, written by Robert Lewis Stevenson:

> "A birdie with a yellow bill
> Hopped upon the window sill,
> Cocked his shining eye and said:
> Ain't you 'shamed, you sleepy-head?"

Or lines written by Milton, the blind poet:

> "To hear the lark begin his flight,
> And singing startle the dull night;
> From his watchtower in the skies,
> 'Til the dappled dawn doth rise."

BOOKS

Discover reading backgrounds of those in your care. Are they mystery, romance, science fiction? Do they need large-print books and magazines? Locate the source for these and for books on tape. Inquire at a local blind center or call the public library. Allow individuals to have a few favorite books in room. Develop a library accessible to persons in a personal-care facility. Wheel a book caddy from room to room on a regular basis. Provide volunteer readers to an aged person who had always loved books. A child or teen can benefit, too, by being a reader. Recognize suggestions from residents. A nursing home resident, following a seed-planting activity, called her daughter to bring the story of "Jack-in-the-Bean-Stalk" on her next visit. Three dog-eared children's books were produced and read aloud as beans planted in a cup were inspected, measured, and placed again on the window sill.

Locate individuals who will give book reviews.

Provide best lighting possible and even a magnifying glass to individuals who are readers. Of all nursing home residents the individual lover and reader of books is least lonely of all.

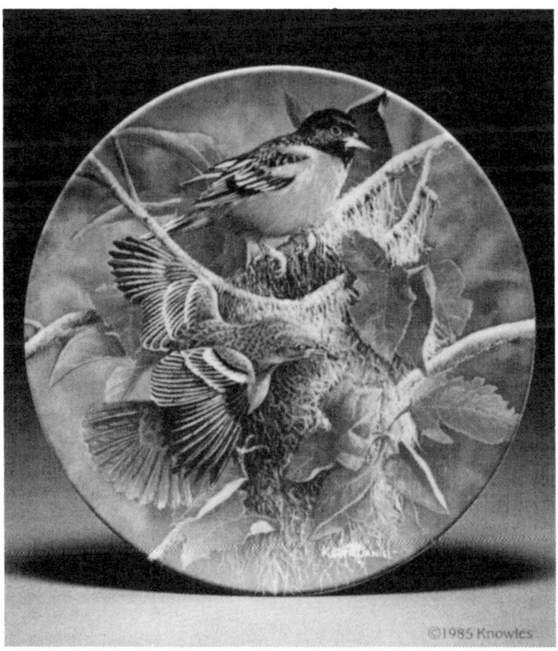

C

CHILDREN
CRAFTS
CURRENT EVENTS

CHILDREN

Caregivers who will provide opportunity for elderly persons to enjoy children can be assured that maximum joy and delight on part of both the elderly people and children will result. Enlist young parents who feel house-bound to visit a nursing home, especially if their parents are far away and both parent and child can benefit from visiting shut-ins. Make list of nursery schools, kindergartens, et cetera, and solicit early from the teachers a time to bring children to visit. Holidays such as Halloween, Valentine's Day, Christmas afford activities that benefit both children and older adults — making cards, wearing a home-made mask for halloween, delivering valentines, and hand-made Christmas gifts. Good attitudes, appreciation each for the other, and lessening of fear are a few by-products of intergenerational activities.

CRAFTS

Know your clientele when planning a craft time and plan for maximum ease of participation in each activity. Craft activity may be welcomed or unwelcomed. A person's attitude or response to participation in an activity is influenced by agility and dexterity. Hands and fingers may not manipulate well. Also diminished sight and other physical factors that accompany age limit ability to participate. Another factor influencing a person's readiness for craft activity may date back to a time when he/she failed to achieve the end product expected. A participant may still feel that perfection is required, whatever the end product. He/she may have been given a pattern to draw, or been confined within lines, or judged on neatness. Such directions are stifling at any age and such critique contributes to a defeatist attitude of 'I can't". The recalling of "failure" comes at the thought of arts and crafts.

Evaluate the following craft activites for their suitability to one for whom you care, or for use in a group.

TREE DECORATIONS: Paste seals on dyed or plastic eggs. Cut flowers from seed catalog to pasted on circle, square, or triangle cut from colored paper of the individual's choosing. Punch holes, thread with ribbon, tie. Loop over tree branches for a spring time tree. Have each participant place a decoration on a tree. This can be a Christmastime activity. Make a winter bird feeder with suet, netting and string. Hang on an outside tree. Watch for a cardinal or chickadee.

PICTURE PAINTING: Try painting a picture on paper with rubber cement. Brush the paper with a thin coat of water color. When the paint dries, rub off the cement. Make a sample to demonstrate.

VASE MAKING: Coat a bottle or jar with white glue. Wrap it with yarn, ribbon or ric-rac. Shellac if desired. The result will be a pretty container for flowers, artifical or real.

POMANDERS: Turn an orange, apple, or lemon into a good smelling pomander. Stick whole cloves into the fruit. Wrap it in a piece of netting and tie with a ribbon. Hang in a closet. The aroma gets sweeter as the fruit dries.

"HAND" MADE WREATH: Trace around hands using green paper. Cut out and glue hands touching each other to form a wreath. Add a red bow. Nice for a Christmas bulletin board. Personalize by signing names either on each hand or add small caption with names of each one who participated in making the wreath.

FAMILY TABLE CLOTH: Start with an old sheet, or tablecloth, or yards of heavy cotton fabric, any color. Supply multi-colored marking pens or crayons. Let each individual *doodle* on a corner of the cloth. Practice *doodling* on a piece of paper first. Scribble a design, do tic-tac-toes, draw happy faces, or a flower, or do your signature. If there is a person who embroiders, these designs might be embroidered with floss for a more permanent product.

AUTUMN CENTERPIECE: Here are step-by-step directions for this group activity:

1. Play music to set autumn mood as residents gather.

2. Give persons opportunity to look over items assembled on trays: pumpkins, gourds, dried flowers, leaves, corn stalks, nuts, apples. Craft supplies: glue sticks, felt, construction paper, scissors, magic markers, et cetera.

3. Identify the task: to arrange a centerpiece for each nurse's station, using a tray for the base.

4. Demonstrate a centerpiece. Show Japanese-style of arranging with tall, medium, and low masses representing heaven, man and earth.

5. Begin work in small groups. Each small group working as a team will function differently; some resisting, doubting while pondering, thinking, selecting items, and eventually creating a satisfying end-product — a neat project with a totally surprised clientele, happy with their creation.

Remember when working with individuals whose mobility and dexterity is limited, prepare as you would for a kindergarten class. When paints are being used have an apron or covering so the individual is free to splash. Be sure the work space is adequate for accomplishing the task.

CURRENT EVENTS

Today television covers happenings across the world two and three times a day. A television is found in every hospital and health-care facility room. Daily newspaper and weekly news magazines describe in depth what passes quickly over the tube. Keeping abreast of what is happening in the world, keeps persons of any age in touch with realities.

Consider the value derived when a small group talks about these happenings.

A special current events program-aid, called "NEWSCURRENTS" could be a part of every health-care facility's program. Write to *"Newscurrents"*, P.O. Box 52 DNK, Madison, Wisconsin 53791-9438. Ask for information about the 35 week, 24 frame color filmstrip and discussion guide. Cost: Approximately $275. with possible free filmstrip projector with a first year subscription. This valuable resource promotes reality orientation, provides news on a timely basis, and stimulates social interaction in addition to being easy to use.

D

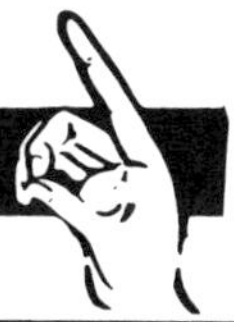

DANCE
DEATH
DOLLS

DANCE

Music prompts the body to move in response to the beat that it hears or feels no matter how young or old that body. Every culture has sacred dance and related rituals. In America, new dance forms are born which characterize an era: The Charlston, the Waltz, Cha-Cha, Swing, The Boogie. The love of dance does not pass away with age or infirmity.

Plan a dance. Begin by assembling a group to talk about dance, dance partners, dance music, dance events — hops, jams, proms — square or country dancing, Arthur Murray and ballroom dancing. Listen to the response each makes. Next, select a committe to plan a dance program. You may find a resident who has been a dance instructor, or a disc jockey. Many persons played an instrument when they were younger. Someone has good ideas for decorations and refreshments. Only after the committee has planned should help be solicited to execute the plan: issue invitations, locate the music, and assist with the setting — low lights, decorations, refreshments. A camera to capture the event plus a newspaper reporter completes the plan.

Other programs might feature American Indian, Hawaiian, or Mexican culture. National groups that work to keep alive their traditions of food, dance, stories — Irish, Scottish, German, e.g. might be invited to demonstrate their dances. Their leader may encourage persons to sway, tap foot, clap hands or move head while using a walker or sitting in wheel chair.

DEATH

Ginny, a strong-spirited double amputee, with marginal sight loved to play Bingo. Margaret who lived across the hall became a real friend. She played Ginny's card for her. Bingo players remember the day Ginny found a special role to play. She surprised everyone by echoing the number being called by the person directing the game. Those having difficulty hearing welcomed her strong voice. Her spirit inspired many.

The day Ginny died, Margaret sat alone in the hall outside Ginny's room. A volunteer who just learned of Ginny's death spotted Margaret, went to her. They shed a few tears together. "We will miss Ginny. Our lives are better for knowing her." The story can be repeated again and again in the long-time care facility.

Who in a busy health-care facility is responsible for allowing a time of mourning? Is the death of a resident treated as a routine happening? Many elders living out their years in a long-time care facility, have come to terms with death. Facing their mortality began much earlier in their lives. Teachers had students memorize writings such as Longfellow's "Psalm of Life" or Tennyson's "When Earth's Last Picture is Painted."

Locate some of these poetic works related to life, death, and immortality. Bring persons together to read, recall, and find satisfaction in sharing life's deeper meaning together. Observe that the residents' reading of obituaries in the daily paper is essential. Sharing stories about the deceased individual brings a satisfaction that tribute was given to that individual.

Know what goes on in the grieving process: guilt, anger, denial, acceptance and moving on. Each individual deals with one or another aspect of grief at one time or another. A chaplain, priest or pastor may be there to allow any of these expressions of grief. Can you help a grieving family find a moment of comfort? Have you faced your mortality? Talk with a pastor/counselor about ways. Explore opportunities to train as a hospice volunteer, to serve terminally ill individuals. Ask your local hospital to direct you to this program.

DOLLS

Visit a health-care facility and note at least one person holding a doll. Family and friends frequently surround their loved one with stuffed animals and dolls.

A Doll Festival in a nursing home might be simply negotiated. Invite persons to bring a doll to the festival. Encourage each individual to tell about his or her doll. Seat persons in close enough proximity that dolls can be passed one to the other to see and to touch. A Doll Festival might be shared with a kindergarten class who comes to visit, each bringing a doll to show, even as residents show their dolls to the children. Talk about the doll's characteristics: bisque head, moveable joints, et cetera.

At another time, invite a guest whose hobby is making dolls, or a seamstress who dresses dolls. Some doll hobbyists concentrate on certain themes, for instance dressing dolls to represent first ladies, or dolls of the White House. Patterns for dressing dolls in blue and gray, to represent Civil war, North and South, are used in one doll-making class. For persons who have no grandchildren dolls and doll-making fill a deeply-felt void.

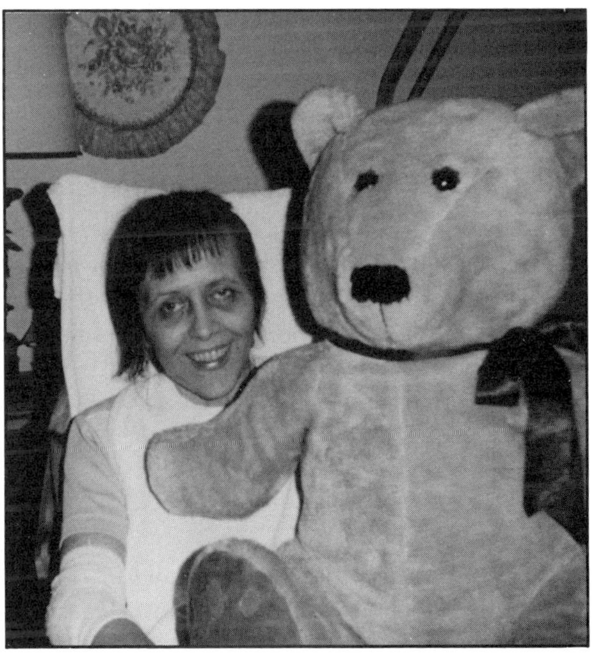

E

EDUCATION
ENERGIZERS
EVENING
EXERCISES

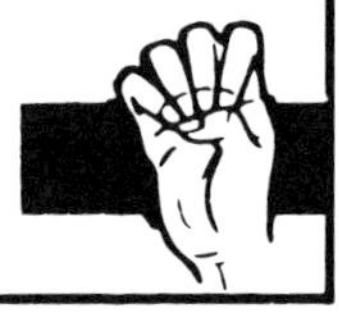

EDUCATION

Elderhostel, an education program for older adults who want to expand their horizons and develop new interests began in 1975 and yearly enroll some 190,000 persons in programs in fifty states, ten Canadian provinces and in forty countries overseas. Usually three minicourses are offered each meeting three- or four-times in the week-long program. Each course is taught by a skilled instructor from the sponsoring college. Participants are free to choose what they would like to do throughout the week.

Plan a *mini-elderhostel* for your facility.

First, canvass residents asking the question: If you could go back to school, what would you like to learn? Compile responses. Give them a list of possible subjects from which to chose. (Popular at Elderhostels are: history pertinent to the area, the culture of a group of people, music or story-telling native to the area where the Elderhostel is held, how-to classes such as making maple sugar or paper, the world of nature, and how to write your own story). Choose your "curriculum" and enlist a presenter for each subject. Schedule a time each day for five days. List the classes to be offered and enroll residents. Award a certificate to each one who has completed the five different half-hour to forty-five minute classes.

ENERGIZERS

"An *energizer* a day keeps the doldrums away." A visit to the hair-dresser, the barber, the manicurist and pedicurist — each restores dignity and pride and should be regularly scheduled and facilitated for the aging person. Any personal grooming, even shining shoes, makes for a good feeling about one's self and one's relationship to his/her world.

A visit from a child, youth, or special family member or friend brings zest and renewed energy to a person confined to a home, be it one's own or a nursing home.

Changes of scenery, visits away from home, lunch with friends, and any number of activities in which individuals may participate eliminates boredom and wards off potential depression. Something as simple as a surprise letter or package may serve as an energizer.

EVENING

Plan to watch a sunset. Sit under the stars for a half hour before retiring. Identify star formations. Look for the Aurora Borealis and shooting stars in a summer sky.

Compile a list of evening songs, psalms, poems to share.

Remember the years of childhood when you were tucked into bed? Or when you quieted your children before they would go to sleep? Why not continue to have an evening conversation with the elderly person for whom you care? Talk over the day's happenings. Have a good-night prayer together.

EXERCISES

Consult with the YWCA or YMCA or local Wellness Center about appropriate exercises for the person under your care. Ask for someone to speak to a group on the importance of exercise, and demonstrate a daily or semi-daily routine each can do in his or her own room.

Special tapes with exercise directions for persons confined to a wheel chair are available. These tapes give directions to exercise hands, arms, fingers, ankles, and legs. Stimulus given to each part of the body improves circulation which in turn helps each person feel more alive and interested in the world around him/her. See section on *Useful Information* for catalogs which contain the source for these aids.

F

FAMILY TABLE
FAVORITE THINGS
FLOWERS
FINGER SPELLING

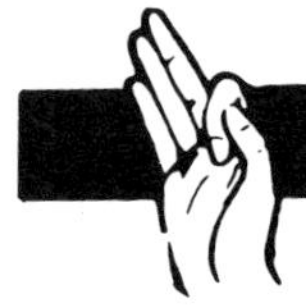

FAMILY TABLE

The subject of the family table is a good conversation starter with the elderly one you are visiting, perhaps for the first time, and from whom you want to glean some information. To prepare for a conversation consider your own family table. What was it like? Who sat around it? If you were to color it, would it be a warm color, cool, cold, hot? How would you color those who sat at the table? How would you color yourself?

The following is a response of one elderly person, when asked that question: "There were eleven of us. I was the baby. Two of us were in highchairs. Benches were on each side of the table for the boys. Mother sat with a highchair on either side of her. Father minded the boys. It took a lot of food to feed that family!" Many an interesting story followed — driving a buggy to the station to meet father's train when he came home from work, the country store, and feelings about family members.

FAVORITE THINGS

Who does not have "favorite things"? Make a time for grandparents to share with family members some of his/her favorite things. (If that individual needs to make transition from his/her home to a special care facility keep a list and locate some of his/her favorite things to have in the new setting.)

To begin a program with a group on favorite things show a portion of the video: *Sound of Music* where Julie Andrews teaches the vonTrapp children the song, "My Favorite Things." Sing it. List favorite things named by each individual. Weave these favorite things into a song. Keep the list and surprise each "owner" of "a favorite thing" with that thing if in some way it can be provided.

FLOWERS

Flower and seed catalogs arrive in the mail in early February. Use them to the fullest. Direct individuals to look through the catalog. Imagine a summer garden. Choose flowers one would like to order. If possible with family cooperation bring the plans to reality.

When finished with the plan for summer garden, cut out pictures to make a collection of favorite flowers. Paste each on an index card.

A collection of cards can be used in many ways. A person confined to bed might enjoy flipping through them for sheer enjoyment, or arrange them in alphabetical order or by color.

Use them for a spelling bee: Coreopsis, crocus, jonquil might be spelled or identified by color or other description. One ninety-six year old flower-lover identified every flower named in the catalog. Locate the piece of music: *"An English Country Garden."* Enjoy the flowers named in it. Add ideas of your own or invite a florist to talk about ways to raise healthy flowers, or demonstrate making a corsage. Have a flower-arranging class.

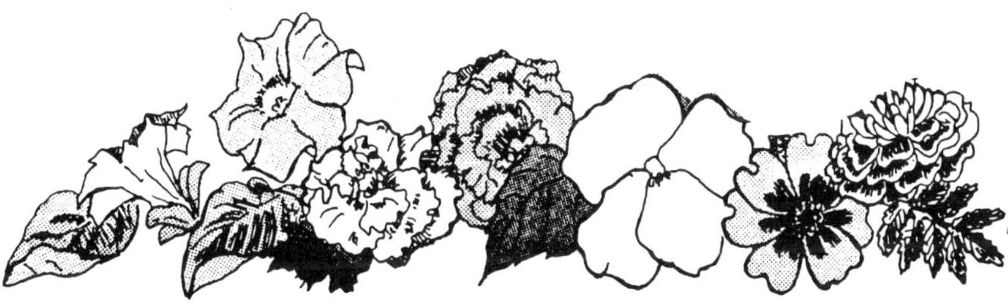

FINGER SPELLING

This activity emerged when numerous senior centers asked how they could help participants com-

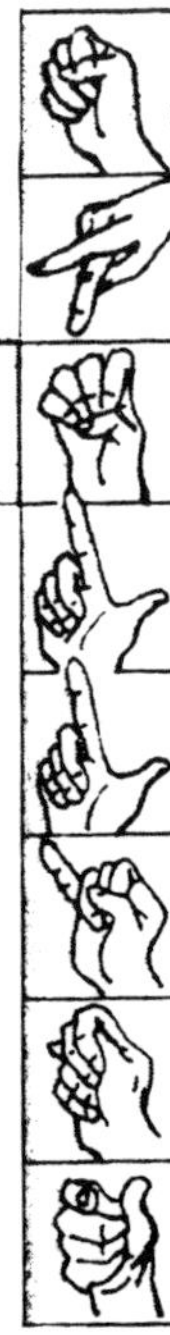

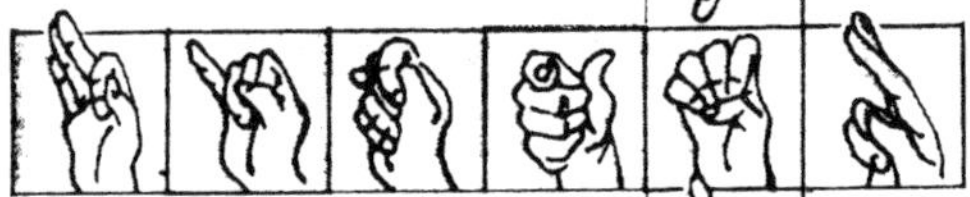

municate with other persons in their group who were having hearing problems.

The activity necessitates learning the manual alphabet. See Appendix. Provide a copy of the alphabet for each individual to study at leisure. Heed simple rules: keep palm facing out; spell letters in place; don't bounce around; aim for smoothness; say words as you spell them. When individuals have mastered it fairly well, seat partners across from one another. Have a page of three-letter words; e.g. *bat, ban, bar, bed, bad, bud, bit, bin, boy, can, cat, cab, cap, car, cot, coy, cup, cap.* Partners take turns finger-spelling a word to the other — alternate "sending" and "receiving". In addition to the intrigue of learning a new language this activity keeps fingers and hands limber, mind agile and alert, and enhances communication. For persons who have difficulty getting to sleep practicing the alphabet can be a relaxing exercise.

Finger-spelling leads to learning simple signs with which to communicate — a beginning understanding of American Sign Language. See Appendix.

GAMES
GARDENING
GROUPINGS

GAMES

The following are a few simple games chosen to use after the evening meal to fill the longer daylight hours, and forstall the desire to retire early.

BALL BOUNCE. Bounce ball from seated position so it will land in a wastebasket or box. Score ten points for each ball that goes in. Give three tries. Double the score if all tries get in the container. Use a knitted ball stuffed with styrofoam. Place chairs in semi-circle with basket equal distance from each seated player. Conclude with basketball stories. This activity can take place on a porch or patio at sunset time.

COLOR IN A BOTTLE. Assemble fruit-juice bottle or Mason jar and box of kindergarten-size crayons. Assign a point count to each crayon; e.g., red-10, yellow-9, black-8, et cetera. Set distances and heights for dropping crayons in bottle so participants can score points. Take turns. Keep score of each. Recognize top scorer.

RING THE CHAIR LEG. Turn a chair upside down. Mark each leg with count; e.g., 5, 10, 15, 20 points and 50 if each of four rings are successfully placed on chair legs. Use Mason jar rings.

LAWN GAMES. Croquet and lawn bowling are appropriate for those who need more activity after supper on a summer evening. Patronize garage sales for good used sets of the above. Outdoor shuffleboard and miniature golf are other possibilities.

GARDENING

A basket full of bulbs, a spade full of soil, a selection of seeds, something as simple as a tin can, an egg carton, a styrofoam cup, a watering can, and a bit of fertilizer are needed for this activity to transpire around a kitchen table. Planting seeds and watching for growth is probably the number one activity that separates those who have and those who have not ever put their hands in the good, cool earth, and rubbed the planting soil through their fingers.

Planting beans is an easy activity in a nursing home, requiring soil, seed, bit of fertilizer and cup. Residents can watch to see how much they grow each day. One resident nurtures her plant along until it actually has three small string beans on it — a miracle in a bedroom window. Flowers can be started indoors as can some vegetables with the aid of special lights. They can then be transplanted out of doors. Retirement centers will have garden plots where residents can grow both flowers and produce. February through May are the best times to schedule a gardening activity.

Since flowers carry with them signs of love, locate individuals who are alone and see that fresh flowers are taken to brighten a day.

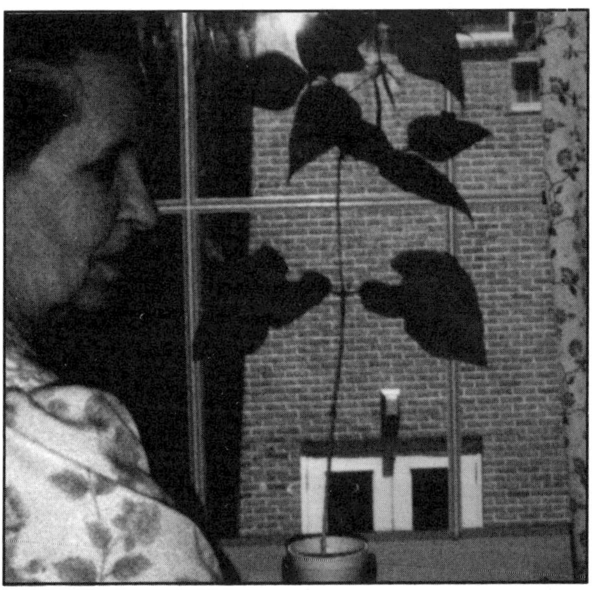

GROUPINGS

One finds among residents in any facility wide diversity of personality, state of health and ability to perform or participate in group activities. The planner of an activity should remember that each participant deserves to find satisfaction in the program planned. Some residents are patient with their peers, others impatient. Others are timid, unsure of self and bodily disfunction. Yet others cannot feel safe trying something new. Some may recall an unhappy experience.

Place a helping person with one who needs assistance. Place a volunteer at a table with four or six residents. The stimulation of an outsider can be good for some, not good for others. A constantly critical resident placed with a gentle, kindly, soft-spoken person may if given time temper each other.

Skilled nursing-home staff place roommates knowing that one can enhance the well-being of the other, or negate it.

The married couple, each needing assistance with living tasks, while not in the most private setting in a nursing home live as normally as possible in the midst of a facility where they can get help they need and at the same time satisfy their own personal desires.

It is best that couples room separately when each one needs specialized care. Time is made for periods together, mealtime or a morning hour, and when family comes to visit.

There are occasional affections that blossom romantically between two persons who have lost their spouses. A wedding is held in the nursing home, and sensitive staff aid family and the new couple in setting up new living arrangements in the nursing or retirement home. The Sweetheart Party held annually in one facility began with a wedding and continued yearly near St. Valentines' Day.

Dining groups are important too, and are as vital as the food enjoyed together. Trust individuals to find those whose company they enjoy, and allow them to build friendships, while accepting the wide diversity around them.

H

HISTORY
HOUSE AND HOME
HUMOR

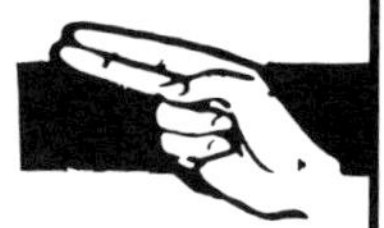

HISTORY

Many persons now living in personal care or nursing homes have lived through more history than students master in school today. Schedule a monthly history program, selecting an era from the late 1800's through the Watergate or Irangate scandals and the hearings to confirm a Supreme Court justice. Focus on the politic, music, major events of a chosen year, or four years or a decade. The recall and mental stimulation that accompanies such a program is extremely beneficial to the continuing well-being of each participant. Other possibilities; choose themes through history; e.g., political conventions, slogans, wars, people in Black history, statehood, national park acquisition.

HOUSE AND HOME

For the new resident in any facility the subject of house and home may yet be filled with the pain of separation. If the resident is placed in the facility following removal from home to hospital to nursing home, circumventing any part of the decision-making process, temporary or prolonged disorientation can result. Preparation for such a move begins in an individuals own home calling for others in the family to participate in looking ahead.

Out of a comfortable home in a Pennsylvania village and into a Jacksonville, Florida retirement center, one lone woman found herself in a small apartment on the seventh floor with a beautiful view of the bay, bathed in morning sunrises and dotted with twinkling lights of ships coming and going — a spot her son felt ideal. He went north, gathered some of her furnishings and set up her new apartment. After watching the view for a week, and wondering why she did not have some of her favorite things, she was a most isolated and miserable person.

Activities that help individuals face the end of a chapter and the beginning of another are essential. Other conversations might center on favorite rooms in the house, or places I have lived. Stories — happy and sad — either way help one accept the present reality.

HUMOR

Correspondent and author Norman Cousins at one point in his life had to deal with life-threatening arthritis. In his book *Anatomy of an Illness as Perceived by the Patient* he details his recovery through a regimen of vitamin C and well-rounded doses of good humor. Thus, all of the *Abbott and Costello* and *The Three Stooges*, films were "consumed" again and again.

Listen for good humor stories relayed among residents. Shortly after the 1988 election of George Bush to the presidency, there echoed the lament: "The White House will have no Christmas tree this year." "Why?" one innocently asks. The response: "There will be only Bushes."

Plan ways to keep a sense of humor alive. Schedule film afore mentioned. Have a *George and Gracie* program. George Burns soon will reach the age of one hundred and is still performing. His poignant routine of visiting Gracie's burial place to have a conversation assures many elderly widows and widowers "It's all right to keep in touch." Caretakers need to recognize that it's all right to laugh and have fun, in fact, it is therapeutic.

Video tape a Bob Hope show and present it at a time when residents might gather in the TV room to watch it together.

Assist residents in planning their own show. Videotape it. Some might contain such old chestnuts as "The Tale of Two Frogs" who fell ker-plunk into a can of cream. One frog said, "It's all over now" and soon it was. The other frog did not give up but continued to kick violently. He kicked and splashed until the force of his kicking churned a big lump of golden butter. Hopping upon it he rode the buttermilk waves to triumph.

I

INTERGENERATIONS
INVENTIONS
INVITATIONS

INTERGENERATIONS

Relate to a near-by public school, or a teacher in that school. Children might visit a nursing home taking valentines, May baskets, show Halloween costumes, begin an adopt-a-grandparent program. Take a few elders to visit a modern-day classroom to talk with children about a one-room school and their early education experiences. Hold a spelling bee, showing children what good spellers some of our older friends are. Have children write stories, interview an octogenarian.

Children and grandparents are good, game players. The family members in the middle of the age span do grandparents and child a favor when they bring out board games, cards, monopoly, scrabble, trivia, checkers and chess. Each enriches the life of the other.

INVENTIONS

The word *invention* itself should prompt many good ideas for a stimulating program to be given in a retirement or health-care center. Develop a BEFORE and AFTER exercise. Many older persons can remember the date many inventions came on the market making a change, small or profound, in their life style. One retirement center planned a word game. The leader with the help of an octogenerian and a teen-ager compiled a list of words to be spelled. One comprised names of tools, et cetera, used before a labor-saving devise was invented. The other listed words such as *lem, fax, VCR*. Seniors expressed astonishment at the number of words to add to their vocabulary and discussed new inventions. Here are the two lists: Yesterday Words: *scythe, hitch racks, bundling, fairy lamp, dry sink, one-hoss shay, cistern, swill barrel, phonograph, schnitz, poll tax, fireless cooker, churn, parlor, out-house.* New in the dictionary: *module, hangar, computer, VCR, remote control, nintendo, aerospace, helicopter, jets, supersonic, transport, lem, fax, television.*

Trace the development of labor-saving devices, transportation, space exploration, disease irradication, diagnostic equipment, et cetera.

INVITATIONS

Recall when you received an invitation. How did you feel? One nursing-home resident had a smile from ear to ear. Excitement pulsed through her body. "I want to ask you a question" she said. "Remember the invitation to attend a party? The party was cancelled because of snow. Tonight my family arrived from Virginia. They are coming to take me out to celebrate. What time must I be in?" Anna was assured she would not be locked out.

Numerous times during a year, a facility will hold a special event to which family members and residents are invited. A personal invitation is often mailed to the family, and residents informed through a public announcement or through the monthly or weekly news sheet.

Consider the value of a personal invitation. Here is a sample invitation to a birthday party:

Dear (insert name):

Congratulations on your (insert month) birthday. You are invited to a party in your honor (day, date, time, and place). Someone will come to get you and bring you back to your room after the party.

If, for any reason you cannot come, please know we are thinking of you. We rejoice in the long life that is yours, and salute you for your beautiful years.

Your friends and persons who serve you at
(name of facility)

A reminder to relatives who have a loved one in a nursing home: Do not overlook that family member when sending invitations to weddings, bar mitzvahs, anniversaries. Remember to send birth and graduation announcements. Indicate to the able individual that you will arrange for him/her to attend the special event. To be remembered is the best medicine.

J

JAM AND JELLY JIGSAW PUZZLES

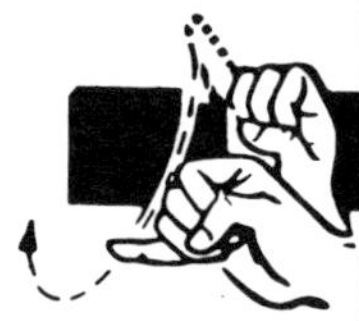

JAM AND JELLY MAKING

Imagine ten or so guests arriving at a place where they are greeted with the aroma of hot baking-powder biscuits just out of the oven. On a table is an autumn display of grasses — an arrangement of wheat and other dried flowers or a cornucopia of apples, nuts and grapes. At one side are some jars of freshly made, sparkly jellies and preserves. Oh, yes, and a crock of creamy butter. Tongue depressor sticks for spreading butter and tasting jellies are nearby. Such an affair could be hosted by a local jellymaker or a homemaker.

Certain locales are the sources of preserves shipped across the country; e.g., Knotts Berry Farms in California and The Country Kettle in Lancaster County in Pennsylvania. Arrange for a visit if one of these is in your area.

MAKE UNCOOKED OR FROZEN BERRY JELLY — Assign guests to be berry cappers, mashers, sugar measurer, jar washer, filler, capper.

Have all equipment ready: large bowls, potato masher, measuring cups, sieves, jelly jars or oleo containers, lids.

NO-COOK STRAWBERRY JAM RECIPE

Stem 1 quart berries. Crush in small amounts.

Measure
1-1/4 cups crushed berries
4 cups sugar
1 CERTO Pectin (comes in pouch)
2 Tablespoons fresh lemon juice

Stir sugar into fruit. Let stand ten minutes. Empty Certo into small bowl. Add lemon juice. Stir pectin mixture into fruit. Stir constantly three minutes. Fill containers. Wipe edges. Cover with lids. Let stand at room temperature for twenty-four hours. Store in freezer.

JIGSAW PUZZLES

Jigsaw puzzles seem to belong in a retirement center or private home, preferably placed where they can remain on a table undisturbed over a period of time, until they are completed. It's nice if a puzzle can be begun by a resident or two and allowed to remain for any who pass by to affix a piece.

Puzzle subjects need to vary. People have different preferences. Some may like abstract designs. Many like a challenge. Puzzles should range from easy to difficult.

THERAPEUTIC PUZZLES. One center for long-term care located a carpenter who glued pictures on pressboard, cut large pieces with a jigsaw and made a frame with raised border into which the puzzle would fit.

A grandmother, blind, palsied, and confined to chair and bed, with the assistance of her grown grandson handled and placed pieces of such a puzzle by tracing with her fingers the open space and the piece she held in her hand.

Another resident, disoriented, confused, unhappy in her new surroundings found solace in a large puzzle. The picture, *The Last Supper* has tablecloth edges, room molding, and the colored garments that serve as guides for placement of pieces. These guides and her familiarity with the picture, enabled her to complete the puzzle with great satisfaction. "We used to do puzzles when my family was growing up" she exclaimed, as a moment of calm and composure came over her.

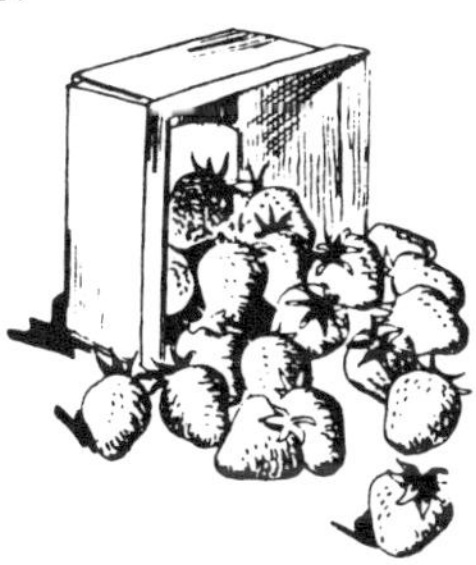

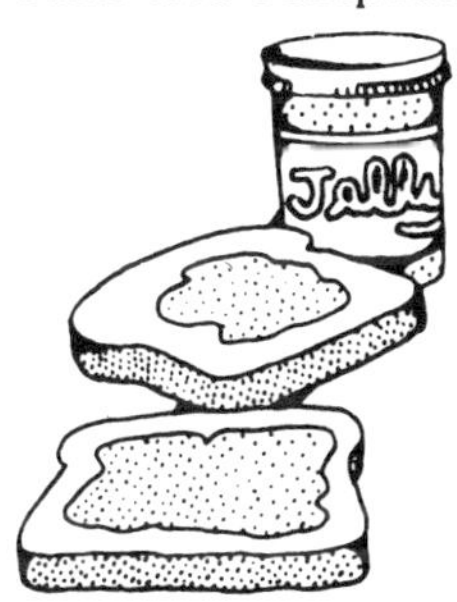

K

KITCHENS
KINFOLK
KNITTING

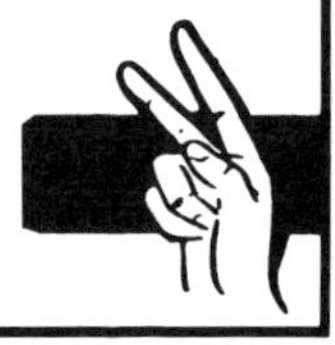

KITCHENS

You can plan an unforgettable afternoon to share with an aging family member in your own home, or hers. Ask an elderly person to describe some kitchens — perhaps a farm kitchen. What kind of equipment did it have? Wood stove, dry sink, icebox? With a series of word pictures trace the evolution of the kitchen. Compare grandmother's kitchen, mother's kitchen, yours, and the transformations that were made over the years.

Invite a representative of a kitchen remodeling firm to bring pictures of new kitchens and describe the modern equipment. Talk about the evolution of the oven. What new life-styles caused fast food industry and microwave ovens to become substitutes for the large family kitchen? Recall happenings in the kitchen — yours, or your mothers. Remember your first cheese fondue that fell before you got it to your guests? And the explosion of a jar while using your oven for canning, and rice that expanded in the pot beyond your wildest expectation. End with a taste of a coffee cake just taken from the oven and a cup of tea or coffee.

KINFOLK

Kinfolk are important to everyone. Genealogies, pages from the family Bible, old newspaper clippings announcing births, weddings, deaths, and legal records, such as deeds to old properties are essential to the completeness of life. Many persons have searched for roots, visited cemeteries, made rubbings from a gravestone containing epitaphs, dates, names, corresponding with persons of the same name, searched archives in county seats, traveled abroad to research a family name. Few have not found this past time intriguing, enlightening, and satisfying.

Such activities on the part of family members lead to the long-term care facility where an elderly member is residing. Assist family members in recording stories that fill in gaps in a family tree. Honor those who were there in the Civil War, the son whose name is on the Vietnam Memorial in Washington, the pioneer woman who with her husband carved out a State in the Union. There are many for whom the Daughters and Sons of the American Revolution are revered for their contribution to family history. Plan a sharing time for residents who would tell you of a famous or infamous member of their family.

KNITTING

Provide those who are knitters with yarn and patterns, that each may continue to be productive. Develop a Knitter's Circle that might meet once a month to show and share and even plan ways to market their wares. Enlist a knitter to teach some children to knit. Recall knitting stockings in World War I to send to the boys overseas, making layettes for the new baby. Make afghans to be distributed to needy persons. Organizations such as Church Women United, Church World Service, or Salvation Army will be happy to assist in delivery of knitted articles.

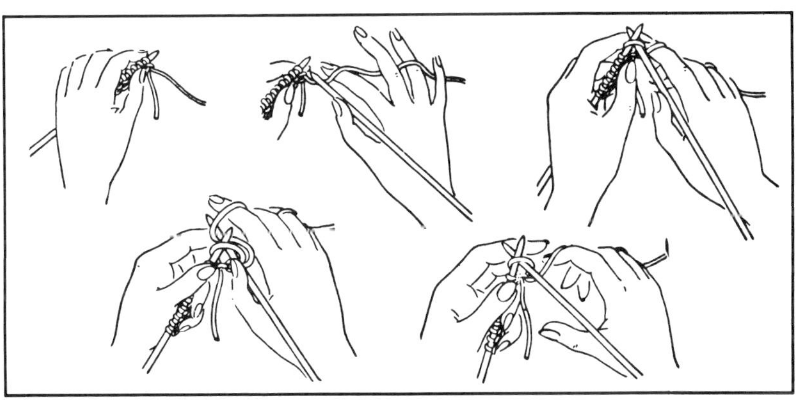

L

LEARNINGS
LETTER-WRITING
LISTENING

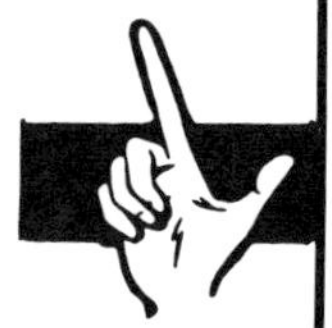

LEARNINGS

"Eureka! I found it!" A piece of information, a skill achieved, an insight or clue. Recall a moment of discovery. How many failures did you experience in the attempt to achieve? A forty-year old recalls her first successful water-skiing experience. Some individuals will tell of learning in the "school of hard knocks". Others claim to be self-taught. That which is now wisdom was first learned, polished and practiced before it could be imparted. It may be identified as one's philosophy of life.

Provide opportunity for philosopher-type persons to gather occasionally for sharing learnings and thoughts on a deeper level. Use a simple starter question such as: What would you like to impart to your grandchildren? Record on newsprint, or tape aspects of the discussion for wider dissemination.

LETTER-WRITING

Many persons who reside in a nursing home need assistance with writing, if they are letter-writers. Sending and receiving mail enables one to keep alert to hours for mail pick-up and delivery. Volunteers who would play private secretary to residents perform unbelievably valuable service. Because of the stimulus of sending and receiving letters one facility for long-term care plans with an elementary school teacher for a letter exchange at the beginning of each school year. Fourth grade children must learn the skill of letter-writing. Names of residents who would respond as a pen pal are sent to the teacher. Each child begins a correspondence with the elderly resident. Unbelievable magic results. Each write frankly and openly to the other. Concerns are shared. It is an experience filled with zest, caring, and sharing even of intimate things. Assist long-lived persons with letter-writing. It can become a lost art.

LISTENING

If you are a caregiver living in close proximity to an aging individual in your home you listen for a bell, a cough, an unfamiliar sound or quiet from that person's room. You listen for feelings noted by the intensity and words that individual is using. You may sense signs that denote depression, fear, confusion, hurt, anger, loneliness, shame, inadequacy. You measure your responses to what you think you hear. You question: "It sounds as though you are . . ." or "It seems as though . . ." or "I feel as though you are . . ." or "It sounds as though you are inwardly disturbed. What is your concern?"

Caregivers and family members need to consider *their* attitudes toward those needing care. The attitude one has influences the ability to really "hear" what is being conveyed. Blocks to listening are many; e.g., *comparing (Aunt Esther always did . . . why can't you), mind-reading (I thought you liked oatmeal every day), rehearsing (Now, if we both approach mother in this . . .), advising (If I were you I wouldn't send that letter), sparring ("It isn't - it is . . .), derailing ("You are making me forget what I was saying . . ."), placating ("I know you feel . . . but tomorrow will be better), topping ("I know just what you mean. Let me tell you what happened to me).*

The blocks to listening might be discussed within a family having difficulty with communication. If you are a caregiver you, too, need to be "as accurately heard" as the one to whom you are giving care. Good listening is a skill to be learned and practiced.

Letters are
A friend's
Best way
To brighten up
Another's day,

And as I write
And think of you
It brightens up
My own day, too!

M

MEALTIMES
MOUNTAINS
MUSIC

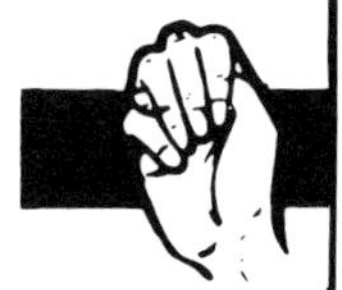

MEALTIMES

Mealtime in America has gone through many changes in the last few decades. The advent of two or more family wage earners, the rise of fast-food outlets and microwave ovens does not lessen the regular three-meal-a-day pattern but eliminates the kind of leisure and fellowship the family table held for previous generations. Mealtime for the aging person living alone or in a nursing home frequently means eating in isolation from some one other than a roommate.

Consider that eating — breaking bread together — with others may be a sacramental act, a holy time, when body, mind and spirit are fed. Note that peoples across the world hold special feasts when the family or community sit down together, eating, laughing, remembering, celebrating life.

In the nursing home that displays the motto: *None shall eat alone*, residents are gathered in small lounges around tables. While they wait to be served, they are directed in singing and conversation. In the personal-care facility, individuals find their way to the dining room to enjoy eating with others. Where there are many unable to feed themselves, a brief time with a volunteer or aide can be warm and pleasant. Mealtime, after all, is that time which orders the day, and should be marked with balanced and palatable foods, clean and cheery surroundings and good fellowship, relaxed and unhurried.

MOUNTAINS

Who knows a mountain?
One who has gone
To worship its beauty
In the dawn;
One who has slept
On its breast at night;
One who has followed
Its longest trail,
And laughed in the face
Of its fiercest gale . . ."

The poet, Ethel Fuller, writing for Dorothy Wells Pease "Altars Under the Sky" (1942: Abington-Cokesbury Press, N.Y., Nashville) communicates with anyone who has loved mountains.

A reading of the above words might inspire the caregiver to develop a program with the theme, Mountains. Pursue a theme of biblical mountains, or mountains to climb and mountain climbing.

Plan time for residents and friends to relate vacation experiences at mountain campgrounds or resorts, and recall taking city and plains visitors to a mountaintop to view magnificent panaoramas.

Conclude a program with the following prayer:

"God of the mountains, hear a mountain lover's prayer. Hear a prayer for courage — courage to face life's problems; courage to meet the unknown; courage to rise above the crowd and heed thy bidding . . .

Hear a prayer for endurance — endurance in the face of storm, endurance over the sharp rocks and crags, endurance to keep on climbing to the end of life's trail. Amen." from Dorothy Wells Pease.

MUSIC

Music is a universal need of the human spirit from the beginning of time. Ralph Waldo Emerson wrote the following:

"Let me go where'er I will
I hear a sky-born music still;
It sounds from all things old,
It sounds from all things young,
From all that's fair, from all that's foul,
Peals out a cheerful song."

He continues by enumerating the places music is found, e.g., in the rose, the rainbow, the stars and even "in the mud and scum of things.

There always, always, something sings. (From "Music" by RWE 1803-1882)

What places might you and the one(s) to whom you give care list as the sources for music using the Emerson poem as a guide?

Music therapist Kimberly Pritchard offers the following understanding, suggestions, helps to caregivers who would provide for maximum enjoyment and participation in creating, singing or listening to music.

"In any environment, there are two basic approaches to music. The first approach uses music as a facilitator to target non-musical goals such as increasing sensory stimulation, range of motion, long-term memory recall and reality orientation. The second approach uses music as the desired outcome to provide positive and reinforcing activies. Both of these approaches, either music as a facilitator or music as the desired outcome, enhance the activity and provide an enjoyable environment.

Various music selections can be chosen for the music-facilitated activity. Often times, familiar music tends to increase the participation level of those involved. Nostalgic recordings provide an excellent aid to activities involving long-term memory recall. Do not hesitate to include "New Age," "Jazz," "Classical," "Country," and "Pop" categories of music. In choosing a selection, be sure to match the mood of the group and then increase or decrease the mood according to the desired goal.

For the production of music as the desired outcome, start a rhythm band using percussive instruments from various locations throughout the world. Latin America provides unique percussion music and may provide an equally unique experience. A chorus is a terrific place to meet and make new friends. In a chorus, start with familiar selections and then increase the repertoire to include newer songs. Encourage an individual to play or sing. Instruments are adaptable to fit needs of the new learner. Practicing not only makes the person play better but requires time out of the day, offsetting boredom and dependence on television. Recitals give everyone a chance to hear how each has improved.

Music enhances wellness, reduces stress and improves the quality of life for anyone who is involved either actively or passively. Music is used to induce response from dimentia and Alzheimers' patients. "Music is for everyone."

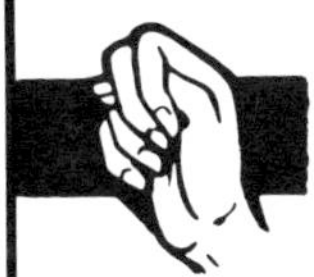

N

NAME ORIGINS
NEWSPAPERS

NAME ORIGINS

"What's in a name?" Expectant parents frequent libraries and pour over a few much-in-demand, dog-eared books of names and name origins. If you have not accessed these for any reason it is worth your time. Explore the history of names: e.g., Lawrence, the potter; John, the smith are names originating from a family trade. Each era will be listed with the most popular names for male and female children, and what influenced the naming of children in that era. Name origins from other cultures may be found in the same book. These will be interesting if you or your elders know Southeast Asians who are neighbors since the Vietnam War. A resident of Italian background coming from a Pennsylvania community can trace family names and similarities to a town in Italy, from which immigrants came who settled the community of Marysville along the river and were the builders of the longest stone-arch bridge.

American Indian names denote a reverence for all of life and strength — Running Deer, Shining Star, Sparkling Water. Explore how names are given in a matriarchal society.

The deaf community select "name signs" which distinguish persons of the same name from each other. The sign may be the placement of the hand in any chosen position on face, arm, or body. Enjoy a group activity where each chooses a name sign. If there is a deaf individual in your center learn to fingerspell first name and then select a name sign. That individual will feel included and participate in other activities with the aid of a few signs.

Any program on name origins should allow participants to tell about their own names. Talk with the "non-communicative" person. Use his name over and over again. Or the constant babbler.

Deep theological and psychological meaning is found in names. Recall the biblical story of the deranged man living among the tombs? When Jesus asked: "What is your name?" his *self* was discovered and his sanity returned. Reread stories of Abram who was renamed Abraham when *he was opened* to great things God held in store for him. Or Simon whom Jesus named Peter, the Rock, when *he grew in his awareness of who he was* and the power within himself.

Remembering that a name is a form of identity, any change of name given to a person at birth creates an identity crisis until the new name is ingested. Married women, feeling the need to keep their identies, take their husband's name but retain their family name. Some years ago, changes were made in the Roman Catholic Church as a result of Pope John's writings. It affected many *women religious* who had renounced their family names to take a saint's name. They were permitted to retake their birth name. For some it caused an "identity crisis." Dealing with this crisis Sister Cynthia Kohler, SCC wrote the following:

He Called Me

"I have called you by name,"
Before the world began to be,
Before the oceans and the seas,
Before the flowers and trees,
He called me.
"I have called you by name,"
Before the angels were formed,
Before mankind was born,
Before Eden's first morn,
He called me.
"I have called you by name."
Before Adam was placed,
Before Eve joined the race,
Before sin brought disgrace,
He called me.

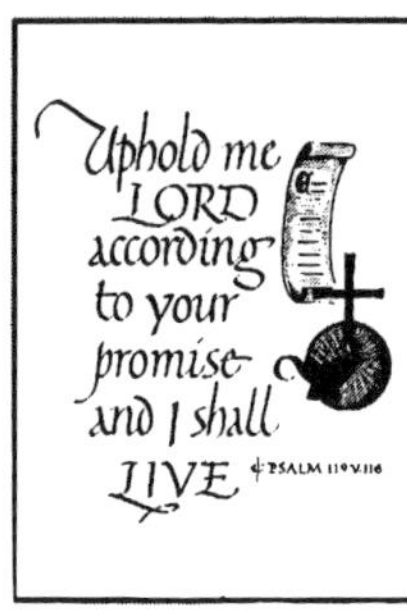
Uphold me
LORD
according
to your
promise
and I shall
LIVE
PSALM 119 V.116

"I have called you by name,"
What love divine!
What peace sublime!
What joy to find
That name is mine!

The name given one at birth is sacred. It should not be taken away. Address persons by the last possession they may have, their name. They revere it. Call them by name.

NEWSPAPERS

Once a newspaper reader always a newspaper reader. While a person whose sight is good prefers to read the daily paper, a scheduled time and place where news is read aloud provides other individuals the opportunity to keep abreast of daily occurences and in touch with reality. Do you know who among older people you take care of would like to receive a daily paper? What can you do about it?

If you are a reader, consider the resident who has difficulty hearing. Provide a device to enhance hearing. Seat those individuals where they can see your face and mouth. Give attention to each section of the paper — sports, comics, obituaries, world, national and local news, and the weather report for the day. Where there are photos, describe them to those whose vision is impaired. Pass that page for the persons with hearing difficulty. Don't underestimate a centenarian whose only extra activity is hearing the newspaper read aloud. "I've always read the daily paper. Why should I stop now?" queries the hundred-and-three-year-old retired elementary-school teacher.

O

OCCUPATIONS

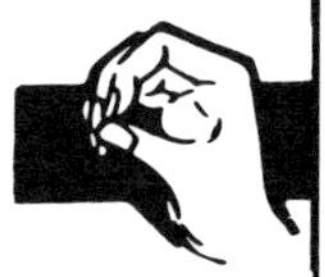

OCCUPATIONS

The dignity of labor and the right to work call most persons to eight-hour days, forty-hour weeks with yearly two-week vacations and provide food for the household, and a work-fellowship with many persons across a life-time. Reflect on the types of gainful employment, and the years of responsible living represented by the lives of persons long retired. Meet the proprietor of a sporting-goods store, the jeweler, the lady cigar maker, a gatherer of sassafras prepared for sale at the market, a proprietess of a local restaurant, a retired director of nursing. Record their stories. Play them to younger generations for persons ready to enter the job market.

The following is a taped conversation with a retired employee of International Paper Company. It illustrates what skill and information resides within the mind and experience of one elderly person who may feel no one cares for his contribution to the world of work.

I. I understand you worked for International Paper Company in York Haven. Won't you tell me about it?

H. I worked there from 1913 to 1960, nearly a half century. I started there when I was thirteen and worked my way up. When I retired I was office manager. Now I am eighty-seven.

I. I'd like to hear how paper is made. You started to tell me when I first visited you. Would you continue the story?

H. You cut logs in four- or five-foot lengths. Try to get spruce and rocket pine. We usually used pine because it would cut into five foot lengths. These go into a machine called a chipper which cuts the wood into slivers. These chips are taken to a steamer where they are cooked for about eight hours with about seventy-five pounds of steam pressure. After that, it is washed and put into vats. Then it is taken to what we call a rut machine. It is bounded and then sent to the beater room. By the way, when I say beater room, that is where the pulp is beat up so it is ready for the paper machine.

The paper is now finished. From there it is put on a wire. This wire travels about five hundred feet per minute, taking the sheet through large rollers which take out all but about twenty-five percent of the moisture.

The paper is now finished and ready for cutting to whatever size is wanted for a master roll.

The master rolls are packaged and shipped. The paper went to Baltimore, New York, Philadelphia, Harrisburg, Lancaster and York.

We used to make the green wrapper for Palmolive Soap. We also made paper for the government. Some of it was called dye wrapping. It went to the Bureau of Engraving and Printing.

I. You have had a great career.

H. By the way, the mill I referred to is demolished entirely. After eighty-five years in service, water power couldn't compete with the big machines run electrically. Now, all that's left is the millrace and trees where people can go and sit in the shade.

One Center chose to honor and affirm their guests for the contributions they made to society. A theme, "End of the Rainbow" was chosen. Brief sketches of the careers of residents were placed in the proverbial "pot at the end of the rainbow" to be read aloud at the appropriate time. In recognition of one's work a ribbon was pinned on each individual. "The Wizard of Oz" folk tale provided music and color.

There are many ways to recognize the worth of work and show honor to the worker. Labor Day may be a good time for such a program in a residence for retired individuals.

P

PARTIES
PETS
POETRY

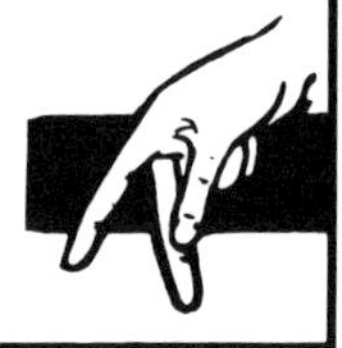

PARTIES

What is a party? Good friends, games, gift-giving? A birthday party is all this and more. Start at the beginning of the alphabet. Each letter begins one ingredient that may be found in a birthday party: *age, birth-date, cake and candles, decorations, edibles, fun and favors, gifts, hands, invitations, joy, kindnesses,love, music, news, old friends, past parties, questions, refreshments, sociability, touch, understanding, visitors, wishes, excitement and years and years of zestful living.* Mix them together and you have a real celebration.

Look in on a nursing-home birthday party. Residents are gathered and seated in a circle. Each is welcomed with a handshake, and a warm greeting from the hostess for the evening. "So happy to see you." A birthday hat and lei are presented to each person having a birthday that month.

A party should have games. Let the games begin. One could be Pantomimes. Each is given a card which tells what to mime. Birthday people go first. Margaret mimes "knitting a sweater". Quickly, others guess. Clyde's act is a push-over. Three persons shout in unison, "starting a Model T Ford" Each guest takes a turn.

Next gift-wrapped packages are passed around the circle to pinch, shake, feel and try to identify the contents. One is eventually given to each whose birth month it is.

A crossword-puzzle book (slightly used) brings a chuckle from Louise. "Someone has seen me with my head in a puzzle book!" she exclaims. Copies of *Workbasket* delight Blanche who exclaims: "For years I subscribed. How did you know I miss it?" Everyone was curious and never guessed that Clyde's gift was a note pad and pencil, in shape of a large mouse with pencil tied to the tail.

Time now for the birthday cake. At the other end of the room tables are set with a centerpiece, candles, placemats, birthday napkin, and a spoon. Dixie cups are in the refrigerator and cakes, made by students from a nearby school, are ready with candles to be lighted.

Guests move to the tables. Lights are dimmed. The glow of two central candles and a small candle on each cupcake, makes each face glow with special beauty. A moment of awe, then the group sings "Happy Birthday." Each person makes a wish, blows out the candle, removes it from the cake and enjoys the birthday refreshments. Another happy birthday evening comes to a close.

Other party resources are:

IMAGINARY GIFTS. Each party guest thinks of an imaginary gift to give. One will suggest a pair of slippers, another might say a plane trip to Disney World, a new car, or a teddy bear. The recipient of each may smile and say "Thank-you."

IMAGINARY GUEST LIST. "Whom would you like to invite to your party?" Ask! Individuals may name family, friends, celebrities, biblical personalities, whomever they can imagine. Record each list to read aloud. A prize may be given to the person with the longest list.

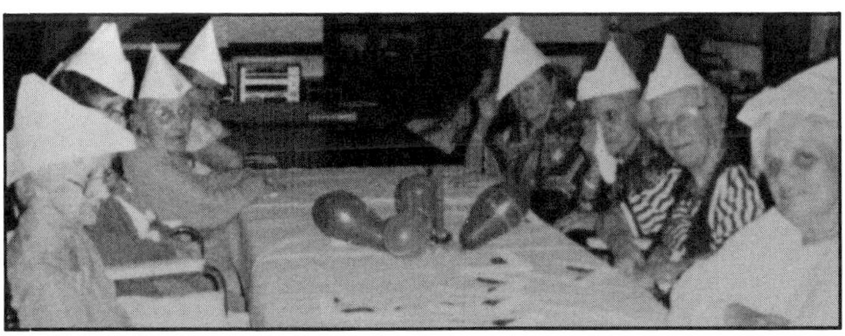

PETS

For seven years, Pumpkin, an orange-colored cat, had been the only other occupant of the spacious house. Its mistress, widowed, with an only son living miles away, found Pumpkin to be a real companion. In fact, so real, that when the widow had to be hospitalized and

Pumpkin taken to board in a nearby animal hospital, daily reports of Pumpkin had to be given to her. There was a problem about what to do with Pumpkin when his mistress found a new residence in a personal-care facility. Her house was sold. Pumpkin went to live in a far away city, and returned once to visit. Months of grieving for the lost pet could only be understood by one who has had a pet and must part with it.

Next, meet Skeeter, a large friendly tiger-marked cat. Skeeter is a permanent resident in a nursing home. He knows little of the outside world except when, on his visits from one room to the other, he spies an open-screened window, leaps up and watches birds in the treetops.

Note what happens when Skeeter walks full length of the table when guests are playing Bingo. Watch expressions on faces and see hands reach out to stroke him. See men and women reach for and cuddle the cat lovingly when Skeeter is taken to visit them.

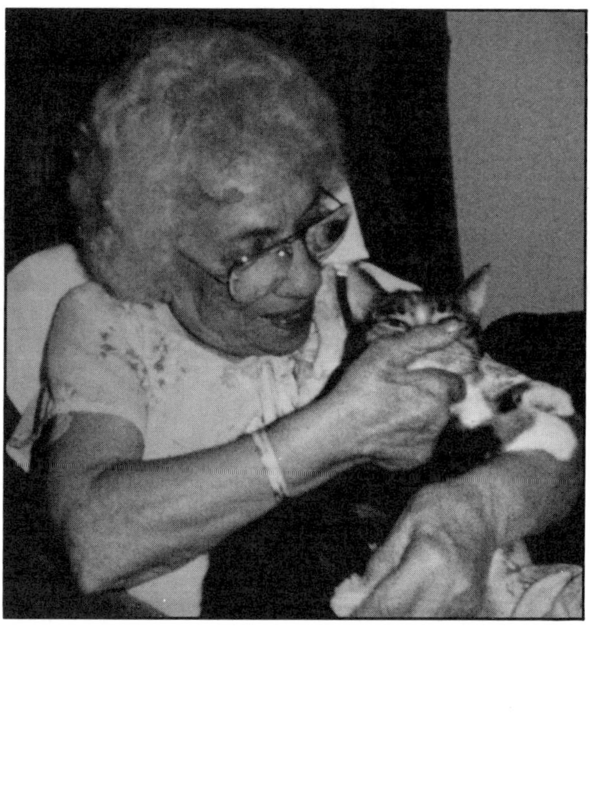

POETRY

Poetry reading is a regularly scheduled activity in many facilities serving the elderly. If you are a poetry reader learn from your audience who are the favorite poets of each one. Discover individuals who have committed to memory works from both American and English poets. Introduce poets that residents have not yet discovered. Recent poet laureate, poets of other countries, ethnic poets, Black and American Indian, young poets.

Search for readings that are humorous and are characterized by alliteration. The latter are fun for the tongue to get around and the ear to hear.

A recording of Robert Frost reading "The Road Not Taken", "Mowing", "Death of a Hired Man" and others can cause the sleepy individual to sit up with a start and listen with rapt attention to the old poet read his verse. Find a local poet. One, Wim Ney, chef in a local facility was readily available. Here is one of his works printed with his permission:

Opus One

"Last night I chopped an onion
slowly and clumsily
my own independent way.
"I fried it in a pan
added an egg
and some cheese
"Memories came back
Strong and pungent like the onion.
Feelings scrambled, like the egg.
Love melted, like the cheese
And held the moment together.
I ate quickly (as you do) and wanted more."

Consider writing some poetry and directing a group in such an exercise. Become acquainted with Japanese poetry, called Haiku. Read and discuss some Haiku verse. Each poem has just seventeen syllables. Five syllables begin a verse and five end a verse. The other seven syllables are in between. Using a chalk board, rewrite a verse separating syllables. Look at them. Count them.

"Spring, unfolds anew . . .
Now in my second
Childhood
Folly, folly, too"

Or

"Within pale silence
Spreading from
Evening moonlight
Suddenly cicada."

Each poem is a picture. Look at the picture in the above poems. Think of an idea and write a Haiku verse. You are painting a small word picture. Now begin one in your group.

Here are directions for writing another kind of poem: Have at hand easel, paper and large markers. Seat persons in a semi-circle facing the easel. Begin by reading some poetry using expression and feeling. Now in a loving, non-threatening atmosphere, laced with good humor, suggest your theme: a favorite color. Select a color named by a member of the group. With that colored magic marker, write B L U E, for example so all can see. Ask how that color makes you feel. Write down expressions from the group. What does the color remind you of? Record responses. Read aloud, rearrange, in poetic form, e.g.;

Blue is my color
It is wide as sky and sea
and as clear as Betsy's eyes
Blue is me when I am sad.
and blue is ice cubes in a glass,
my favorite dress,
and forget-me-nots in summer.

Now read it together.

Have paper and crayons on a table near by for persons to use in any way they like. This type of activity is being tried with persons afflicated with Alzheimer's disease, in an effort to regain some touch with life.

QUILTS
QUILTING

QUILTS / QUILTING

The mention of the words *quilt or quilting* is a generation binder. Today enthusiastic quilters frequent auctions in search of quilts that were created before 1900, and family attics are searched for an heirloom quilt. The treasure tells of a woman's work and recreation, lifestyle, skill, artistic expression.

Some senior centers feature quilting on a regular basis. Start a Quilter's Club. Enlist participants who have made quilts. Listen to stories of quilts they have known. Meet again and look over quilt patterns. Invite a proprietor of a needle-work store or a young quilter of today to bring scraps of materials, pictures of patterns, and briefly tell who is quilting today. Allow time for participants to tell of patterns they used, and the steps in making a simple "crazy quilt." By this time you know the interest and abilities of residents. A third meeting might be to make a pillow top. Find a volunteer who with the help of a resident, will direct this activity bringing needed supplies with her.

At one residence an invited guest told a story as if a quilt were speaking, as she held the quilt in her hand. It went like this:

"Let me introduce myself. I am a piece of each dress made during The Great Depression by a resourceful mother. Each left-over scrap was given to an old lady, who carefully snipped, arranged, stitched and quilted me. She finished as she had planned when she was seventy-seven. I was a gift to her first grandchild on its seventh birthday.

"I will not be forgotten if I and my story pass lovingly from one generation to another. I promise each will find comfort and warmth in knowing how much love and care I hold."

R

READING
RECORD-KEEPING
RELIGION

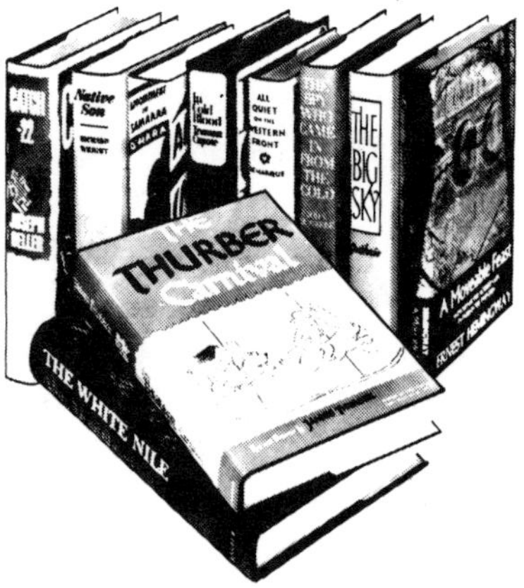

READING

See section on books.

RECORD-KEEPING

Diary-writing, journaling, even recording temperatures and weather have been a daily routine for many retired individuals. One person, Mary by name, a resident in a nursing home, always has with her a little wire-ringed notepad with pencil attached. In it she writes and writes — an idea, a line of a song, name of persons who visit her, the date she sees first robin, et cetera. Praise her for holding on to her personal activity.

The caretaker should be alert to desires of residents to keep writing and supply each one with necessary equipment — notebooks, good pens or pencils and writing boards.

RELIGION

Forget the adage: "Never discuss politics or religion." Careproviders as well as the individual being cared for have rights to their own convictions on both subjects, and may accept or reject participation in religious-type programs.

Religion assists persons to recognize life's movements from stage to stage from earliest childhood to one's last breath; and to affirm life as dynamic, ever growing and changing. Most older persons have moved through stages of maturation that have included asking hard questions, political or religious. Do not ignore either. Since no two persons are alike there may be gaps in growth that need to be filled.

Canvass to see if there is interest in comparing religions. In this shrinking world, television brings into the home cultures other than Judeo-Christian. Invite a rabbi to discuss Judaism. Bring in an Arabic family to visit, and to tell of their traditions, and the characteristics of Islam. A refugee family formerly from Southeast Asia may tell about Buddhism, or an Indian professor from a nearby college might demonstrate Yoga and tell about Hinduism.

Be aware of residents' backgrounds and respect each one. A chaplain or local church pastor who takes time to listen may discover residents who cannot participate in the facility's communion service.

Be cautious of death-bed evangelists, who tend to harangue their audiences. Again know your residents, and respect each personal journey of faith.

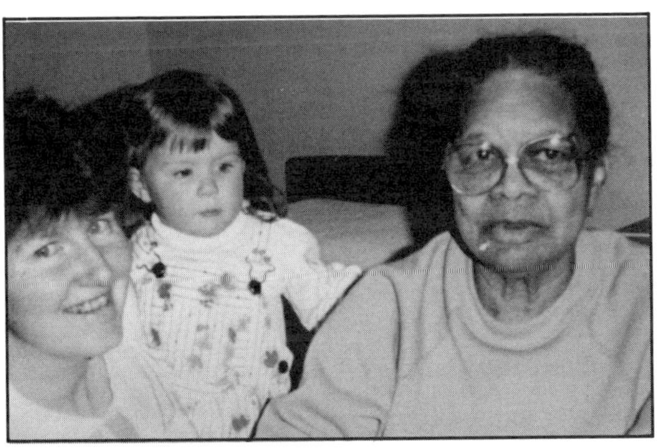

S

SEASONS
SENSES
STORYTELLING

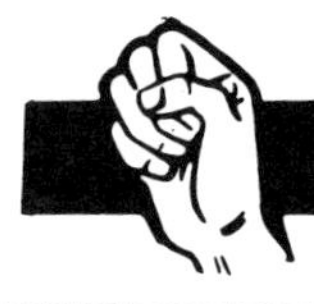

SEASONS

Fall, Winter, Spring and Summer could come and go unrecognized by persons living many years in a long-term care facility. The change of seasons can be marked in a way that helps residents recall different seasons of the past.

Plan a slide program depicting characteristics of the current season. Take a bus tour through farmlands at planting and blossom time. Go to a park in summer to watch swimmers in an outdoor pool or have an outdoor picnic. A Fall foliage tour is always popular.

Locate a group of women who might make a set of seasonal boxes for a nursing home. Shoe boxes, one for each season, are filled with small items that can be handled, smelled, rattled and tasted that characterize that season. Cover the box with paper or pictures to identify the season for which it can be used. A Fall box may contain a miniature football, pumpkin or gourd, ear of dried corn, piece of corn husk, small jars of spice (cinnamon, cloves, ginger)and a package of dried apples. Such a box taken from room to room in a nursing home will stimulate the senses, elicit conversation and renew interest in an otherwise ho-hum day.

SENSES

Sensory stimulation is prescribed by physicians for persons with a variety of illnesses. It is a routine treatment in many nursing homes. Look at activities offered as you visit a facility. Note if *sensory stimulation* is among them. Observe techniques and tools used to stimulate sight, smell, hearing and touch.

Eyes, ears, nose and hands need to be stimulated. The seasonal box described earlier can serve to stimulate each of the senses. Selected activities provide stimulus to the senses. Identify by aroma each fruit placed in a brown bag. Use spices, perfumes and soaps in the same manner.

Taste wine, cheese, jelly and soup. Identify the spice in spicy gumdrops, et cetera.

Listen to bird calls, musical instruments, and house sounds.

Place in each of several bags items to be identified by squeezing and feeling. Think about the hand and what it can do. Join hands around a circle, and play "electricity" by sending a "squeeze" from person to person.

The hug — warm, loving, holding — can ease inward and outward pain, restore energy, and clear tears. Someone has said: *Hugging is practically perfect: No moving parts, no batteries to wear out, no periodic check-ups, low-energy consumption, high-energy yield, inflation-proof, non-fattening, no monthly payments, no insurance requirements, theft-proof, nontaxable, nonpolluting, and, of course, fully refundable.*

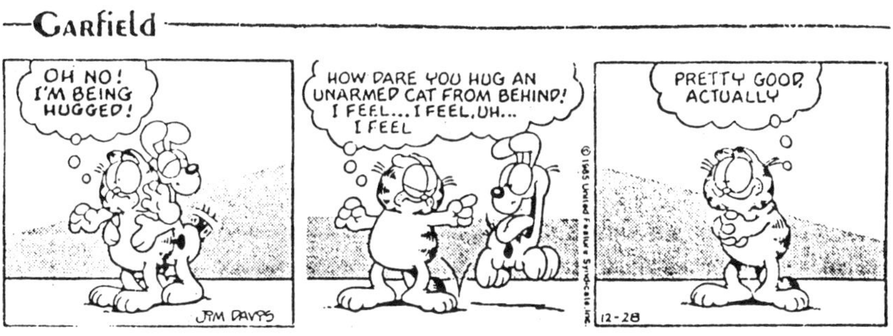
GARFIELD
OH NO! I'M BEING HUGGED!
HOW DARE YOU HUG AN UNARMED CAT FROM BEHIND! I FEEL... I FEEL, UH... I FEEL
PRETTY GOOD, ACTUALLY

Reprinted by permission of UFS, Inc.

STORYTELLING

Recall origins of storytelling: Nomadic people told stories around their campfires which contributed to early biblical records. Jesus was a storyteller. We know many of the parables. "Aesop's Fables" provide a generation with never-to-be-forgotten tales.

The Storytellers' Festival, popular in several parts of the country, successively captures the imagination and delight of creative, imaginative people. Stories such as the ghost of an Alabama fiddler who charmed snakes until he dropped his bow and the snakes killed him. Late at night you can hear the strains of "Amazing Grace" drifting from Fiddler's Ledge. Tales are spun about cannibals, magic eggs, talking donkeys, and peanut, raving catfish and a featherless rooster wearing little bib overalls.

Storytelling needs nothing except a teller and a listener. What fun it can be to sit with a shut-in and together spin some tales. One more suggestion: Create a group story. Start with a sentence and ask each person to add a sentence or happening until all have contributed. Tape the story as it unfolds. Play it back.

Remember every individual has a personal story to tell. Blessed is that individual if you are there to listen. And you will depart with a special gift.

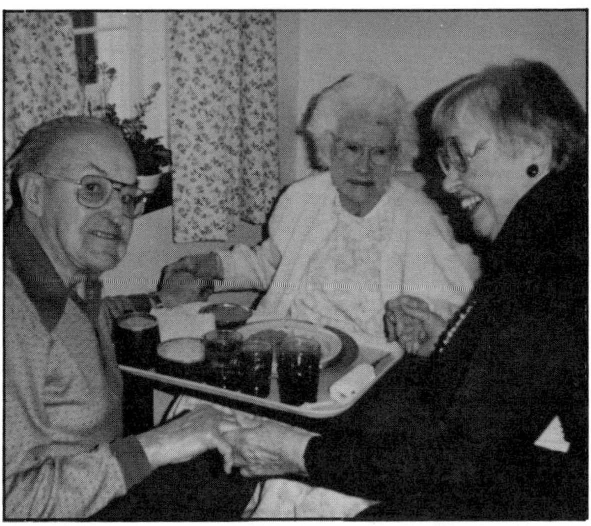

T

TASTING
TOURING

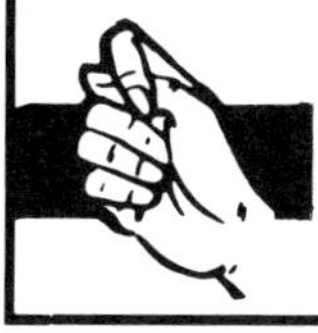

TASTING

With knowledge of the background of elderly people and their dietary restrictions, the following suggestions may be tried:

SOUP TASTING. A local dining room offers on its menu a small cup of each of three soups of the day. Why not a Soup Tasting hosted by a chef who talks about kinds of soups, while preparing one for each to taste.

CHRISTMAS BREADS OR COOKIES. Invite a women's group to meet at a local nursing home and bring samples of cookies to taste. Prepare a recipe that requires little effort to help with by those observing.

WINE AND CHEESE TASTING. Feature a Wine and Cheese-Tasting Party complete with a background of classical music. Arrange a festive setting conducive to conversation and listening. Provide sparkling juices to taste and a variety of cheeses. Few persons in a nursing home are permitted to have alcoholic beverages. Tasting each following the presentation can be an interesting experience. Acquire video or film on wine-making or cheese-making from a local producer.

TOURING

The health-care facility that has a van or bus and licensed drivers is fortunate. The resident who has a friend or family who will take him/her for a short drive to a mini shopping mall, a favorite ice-cream stand, or a pretzel bakery is to be envied. To see outdoor Christmas lights, Spring gardens, a Fourth of July fireworks display is an experience which will be long-remembered, a real bonus to any shut-in able to participate.

U USEFUL INFORMATION

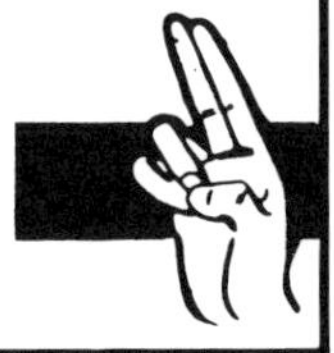

USEFUL INFORMATION

Secure up-to-date information and locate additional resources:

Alzheimer's Disease

Get on a mailing list for a state or national organization, e.g., Alzheimer's Ass'n., South Central Chapter, 600 N. 12th St., Suite 5, Lemoyne, PA 17043.

Call your public library. Ask for book: *Love is Ageless: Stories About Alzheimer's Disease* by Jessica Bryan published by Serola Press.

Interactions By Design, for Alzheimer's programming contains positive interactions programs. There are 50 activities plus a manner of teaching, expanding on what illustrations are in this book. Write Medical & Activities Sales, P.O. Box 4068, Omaha, NE 68104.

Understanding Alzheimer's Disease, $15.95, edited by Miriam K. Aronson, (Scribners, 1988) is for families of Alzheimer's patients. Twenty-six foremost experts discuss diagnosis and treatment, strategies for coping and legal/financial pitfalls. Special sections cover emergency situations, support groups and nursing-home placement.

Stroke and Stroke-care Information

Write National Stroke Association, 300 E. Hampden Ave., Englewood, CO 80116.

For a catalogue offering specialized equipment to promote self-sufficiency, write *adaptABILITY*, P.O. Box 515, Colchester, CT 06415-0515.

Information on Hearing Impairment

Write to *Self-Help for Hard-of-Hearing People, Inc. (SHHH)*, 7800 Wisconsin Ave., Bethesda, MD 20814. Ask for information on ALDS (Assistive Listening Devices) and sample copy of the magazine, *Shhh*.

Ask for *Deaf Patients: a Handbook for Health-Care Professionals*, The National Academy, Gallaudet College, Washington, D.C. 20002.

Information on Visually Handicapped.

The National Association for Visually Handicapped makes available a *Visual Aids and Informational Material Catalog*. Write NAVH, 22 W. 21st. St., 6th Floor, New York,NY 10010 requesting a copy.

Information on Diabetes

Contact your local American Diabetes Association or ADA's Diabetes Information Service Center, 1660 Duke St., Alexandria, VA 22314. The toll-free number is (800) 232-3472.

Program Resources

For slide-tape programs and pamphlets on aging write *American Association Retired Persons, Program Resource Department*, 1090 K Street NW, Washington, D.C. 20049.

The Art of Cooking For the Diabetic by Katharine Middleton and Mary Abbott Hess, A Signet Book, New American Library, 1979, gives recipes for diabetic cooking.

Catalogs for Activity Directors

PICKETT ENTERPRISES, P.O. Box 68, Prescott, AZ 86302
Easy-To-See and Fun-To-Use Activity Supplies

HAMMATT SENIOR PRODUCTS, P.O. Box 727, Mount Vernon, WA 98273
Write for Catalog for Activity Professionals

SEA BAY GAME CO., P.O. Box 162, Middletown, CT 07748
Innovative and Recreational Materials

CRESTWOOD COMPANY, 6625 N. Sidney Place, Milwaukee, WI 53209

Communication Aids for Children and Adults

The following resources may be found in catalogs from one or more of the above companies:

Down Memory Lane by Karras — Topics for Reminiscence Groups.

The Games Older People Play by Lacey

Reality Activities by Cunninghis — A how-to manual to use with confused and disoriented elderly persons

Keep Minds Alert Volume I, II, and III

Parties with a Purpose by Barrett — Parties around the Year

Caregiver Services Beyond Family and Nursing Home

Because of the growing need, in nearly every part of the country, state and local agencies are making available special services of various kinds. Listed below are a few such services:

Adult Day Care. Social contact, a noon meal, and a variety of activities are provided in a supervised setting to persons who due to physical, mental, or emotional problems are unable to be alone at home during the day.

Homemaker Services. Homemaking services assist the individual in regaining and maintaining self-sufficiency through providing personal care. Light housekeeping and laundering tasks may be provided while assisting with personal care. These services provide respite care, enabling the caregiver to leave home for short periods.

Domiciliary Care. Protective living arrangements are made in private homes for disabled adults and frail, elderly persons.

Home Health Care. Visiting Nurses Association makes home nursing care available, often a follow-up of hospitalization.

Escort Services. Transportation vehicles with lifts take senior citizens to social and recreational activities. Escorts may provide supervision to and from doctors' offices.

Senior Centers. A senior center provides balanced activity and noon meal on a daily basis. Some churches offer a similar program on a less frequent basis.

Personal-Care Boarding Homes. This type of home is becoming available as the adult population ages. These homes are licensed and monitored by state departments of welfare. They offer room and board, some supervision to individuals who cannot live independently, i.e., personal hygiene and supervised medication but do not give twenty-four-hour nursing care.

Area Agency on Aging. AAA is a state and/or federally funded office specializing in helping older persons. It provides a broad field of services and helpful information. Locate an office nearest you and write or phone for a listing of their services.

Home Health Care offers a less expensive means of restoring or improving the health of persons with heart, diabetes, cancer or fractures while they enjoy their familiar surroundings and way of life. Locate one of the following services available in your community.

Visiting Nurses Association (VNA). This program provides a nurse specialist to make home visits on a short-term basis. A nurse coordinator of the VNA assesses the need and assigns the appropriate nurse. This program is supported by funds from United Way and other community organizations.

Lutheran Social Services in many regions across the country have a visiting nurse program designed to reach into more isolated areas of a county or state.

Much **useful information** is as near as the telephone. A call to a local city or county Agency on Aging will supply a wealth of information. Many **support groups** meet regularly to share first-hand experiences as well as derive significant educational information.

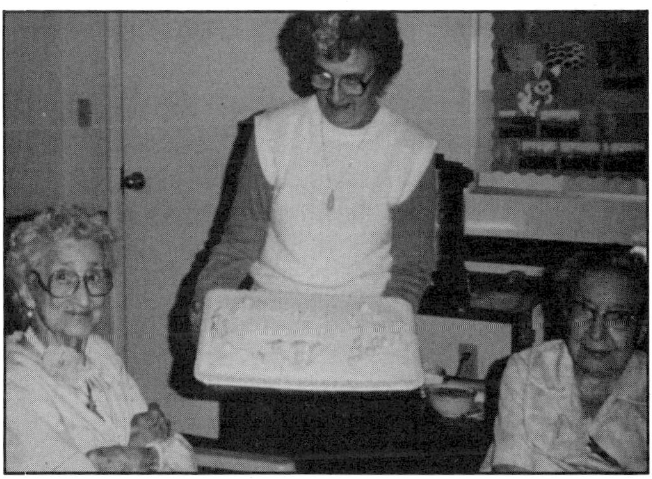

V

VALIDATION
VACATIONS
VISITORS
VOLUNTEERS

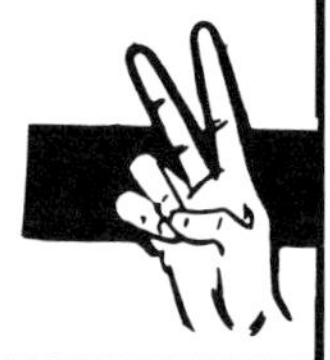

VALIDATION

Validation, a term with specific meaning to therapeutic recreationalists, and staff of long-term care facilities arises from the needs of persons out of touch with reality. You, the caregiver, are called to evaluate the importance of *validating* versus calling to reality the individual who is out of touch, who awaits a visit from her mother whom you know to be deceased. Will you respond: "Your mother was a very special person to you. What do you most remember about her?" To unthinkingly respond with "Your mother has been dead many years. How can she visit you?" is to be less than kind. To skillfully *validate* the confused individual to his/her satisfaction and leave that individual with a calm spirit as opposed to mounting frustration is a recurring necessity when the aging person lives with confusion.

VACATIONS

Canvass clientele to discover vacations they most remember. Where two or three enjoyed the same type, have an afternoon tea time where experiences can be shared

Invite family members to show slides of a recent vacation trip to their elderly person who remained at home, but who followed them in mind's eye being uncertain about their return. Try a program of Imaginary Travel, the kind of vacation you always wanted but never had. Use flat travel pictures, mounted for easier handling, to initiate one-on-one conversation with a shut-in or bedfast resident. Be prepared to listen for a story of an almost-forgotten vacation experience.

VISITORS

Family, friends and church visitors are extremely important to those confined to a nursing home or health-care facility. You may be the friendly visitor to become a care-giver to one whose family lives far away, or who has no family. Acquire names of those who are most alone from the director of a long-term care facility who will assist you with brief orientation to the facility and the individual.

VOLUNTEERS

Individuals who consider making regular visits to a shut-in or resident in a nursing home become an integral part of those serving the needs of either family or institution. Feeding assistance may be needed. Reading aloud, writing letters, taking residents for walks, transporting them to church or shopping are needs to be filled.

Note the following story of how one church group became involved in volunteering. The president of the women's organization started the ball rolling. Members of adult Sunday school classes as well as husbands and children signed up to assist. A part-time employee at a nursing center scheduled each to assist in one way or another. On Sunday afternoons some took wheel-chair residents to the worship hour. Sisters who travel extensively showed slides of a recent visit to Australia and New Zealand. Husbands participated in a craft activity by preparing white branches to be planted in buckets of sand to serve as an Easter or Spring-time tree. Wives and children assisted residents in making decorations to hang on the tree. Others assisted with birthday parties or became regular helpers at Friday evening programs.

Residents quickly related to two recently widowed volunteers and asked about them when they were not there. Little crocheted pins made by one member to represent each month were proudly worn on their sweaters or robe. Months after, a visitor would note the small cross with a pearl in center, or a daisy, a shamrock or a rose.

For many, a hospital or nursing home is a forboding part of an unknown future. Those who draw near to help receive deep and abiding satisfaction, and fears for the future can fade away.

WAITING WONDERING WORSHIPPING

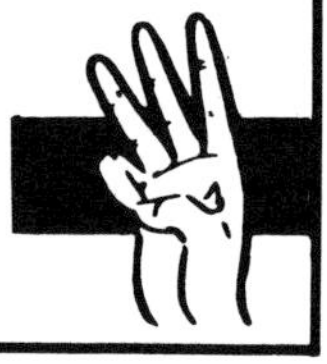

WAITING AND WONDERING

A first-time visit in a health-care facility usually leaves an indelible impression. In a hospital, the ill recover and return to their home, or enter nursing homes to recuperate and/or spend their last days. In the long-term facility reside persons in every stage of life or near death. Who are these persons? Who were they? Why are they here? What do they do all day? What is going on within the mind of these persons?

Waiting, wondering, even *worshipping*, to the visitor may seem the extent of activity for the aging and infirm person.

If you are a caregiver you will be aware of close ties of interminable love going on in the *silence* and *stillness*. Hosts of saints attest to what fills the moments of waiting. Poets and sages have given words to the *silence*. Men and women of faith, tell of the *new future*.

One poet has said:

"Thru the experience of our hearts not our minds, we come alive . . . To be alive is also power . . . Mere existence, even without a further function is "Omnipotence Enough! . . . Every day life feels mightier, and what we have the power to be, more stupendous. A coffin is a small domain yet it is ampler than the sun, and to the one who there bestows a friend it is Circumference without Relief or Estimate — or End — ".

(from "Emily Dickinson" An Interpretative Biography
by Thomas Johnson, The Harvard University Press.)

WORSHIPPING

It is Sunday afternoon in a health-care facility. Those who can be pushed in wheelchairs, walk with walkers or canes, persons who are confused, disoriented and without recall, gather waiting expectantly for the service to begin. Youngest members are those afflicted with multiple sclerosis, AIDS, cerebral palsy. One is a recovering alcoholic. They are Catholic, Protestant, Jew, Assembly of God, Caucasian and Afro-American. The leader of worship begins:

"This is the day the Lord hath made! Let us rejoice and be glad in it." All repeat, then sing: "This is the day . . ." They sign it using deaf sign language.

All bow as the leader prays:

"God, we come today to worship you. We bring you ourselves, our frail bodies and strong spirits. We listen to your Word.We pray your prayer and sing your praise. We hope for new strength. Hear our hearts and heal our thoughts as we continue to worship you. Amen.

A hymn is sung. Mary who knows many hymns leads. A psalm is read. Favorite verses of scripture are shared. Everyone recites the Shepherd Psalm. It is "signed" and discussed.

News of the past week is recounted — a hurricane, an earthquake, a plane crash. Prayers are offered for those who have experienced pain and loss. Someone asks that the song: "God will take care of you" be sung for all those who experience sadness.

The Lord's Prayer is prayed. The group departs after singing "God Be With You Till We Meet Again."

Persons come to the scheduled worship services each week to receive strength for the days ahead.

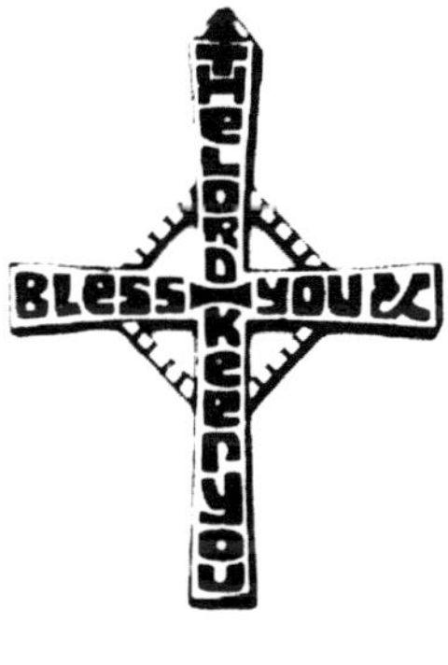

X

XMAS PROGRAMMING

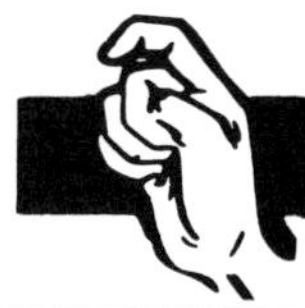

XMAS PROGRAMMING

Much preparation for the celebration and observance of Advent, Christmas and Hanukkah is necessary. Many individuals and groups are needed to make these days significant for residents: tree-trimmers, gift wrappers, decorators, cookie-makers, tradition-carriers, carolers of all ages.

A Hanging of the Greens program, borrowed from YWCA or church may be adapted for residents in a health-care center. Such a program will involve a reader, a narrator, and an individual or group who will place each symbol in an appropriate place as the service proceeds. Christmas carols are interspersed throughout and as many persons as possible participate in giving the setting a festive air in preparation for the season of Advent and coming Christmas Day.

A church group might volunteer to direct the Hanging of the Greens for a nursing home. An innovative teacher might have students do this project, and involve residents to assist.

OTHER DECEMBER ACTIVITIES. Make popcorn balls, simple cookies, and candies. Prepare "goodie plates" to share with others. Residents in a nursing home can do this under the guidance of a staff person, or a volunteer who will come in with the ingredients, and direct the activity.

Assist residents in addressing Christmas or Hanukkah greetings. Thoughtful family members will provide a selection of cards, postage stamps, address list and a gift of "time" to help an aging person continue a life-long custom of sending season's greetings.

Y

YOU

YOURSELF

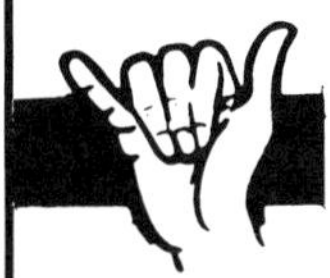

YOU — YOURSELF

An activity dealing with "you"? Why? To help you test whether or not you are ready to be a caregiver. A mother of teenagers, ready to find a satisfying work outside the home was urged to apply for a position in a nearby nursing facility. She would carry water to rooms, aid in feeding patients, deliver mail. She was hired, worked a week and resigned. Better, she reasoned, to give time to her parents, still in good health. "The time will come when I am made ready to serve hurting people beyond my family."

Socrates said "Know thyself." Shakespeare, "To thine ownself be true . . . then follows as the night the day, thou canst not then be false to any man."

Compassion is a necessary quality for a caregiver, and is thought to be a common human attribute. Measure your capacity for compassion. Reflect on those life experiences which heighten that capacity.

Compassion, a word derived from the Latin means *to suffer with*. It call us to go where suffering is, to weep with those who weep. It calls us to be vulnerable, and powerless, with those who are both vulnerable and powerless. Hubert Humphrey was once asked about compassion in politics. Picking up a pencil with an eraser on its end, he responded: . . . look at this pencil. Just as the eraser is only a very small part of this pencil and is used only when you make a mistake, so compassion is only called upon when things get out of hand."

Ours is a society that gives more credence to competition than compassion, to avoiding pain than using it for personal growth, and evading realities through many escape mechanisms.

Measure your "compassion quotient" for being a caregiver.

Z

ZEBRAS
ZOOS
THE ZODIAC

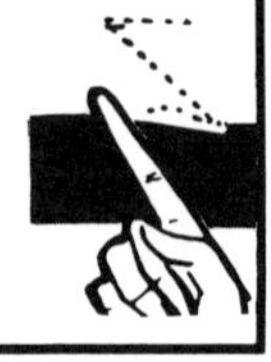

ZEBRAS

Anyone out there interested in zebras? How the zebra got its stripes? Its origin and relationship to the horse? If you find a curious elder in your family bored with nothing to do, provide a volume of an encyclopedia that covers "Z", and let a research project begin. Listen at a dinner table to the findings of the researcher. Anticipate that it could lead, along with children's interests, to a trip to the zoo.

ZOOS

Can you feel the excitement at the very mention of the word zoo? There should not be an elder person who is alive who has not visited a zoo, not a child in a family who could not help push a wheelchair over the turrain of the modern zoo. Let a trip to a zoo be a family affair. If such a visit is planned, inquire about the availability of wheelchairs. Ask if paths allow ease of movement from one part of the zoo park to another. The efforts some quarter-century ago on behalf of handicapped persons assure accessibility to many public places.

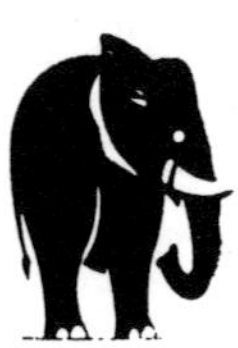

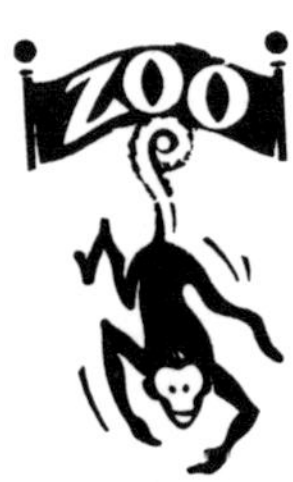

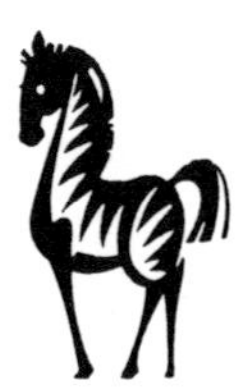

THE ZODIAC

Most newspapers will carry horoscope predictions. While few predictions are pertinent to the individual in his nineties, reading of one's horoscope may continue to hold a residue of interest. Here is a listing for quick reference.

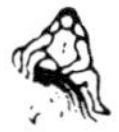 Aquarius . . . . . . (January 21 — February 18)

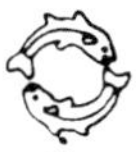 Pisces . . . . (February 19 — March 20)

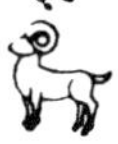 Aries . . . . (March 21 — April 19)

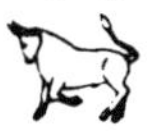 Taurus . . . . (April 20 — May 20)

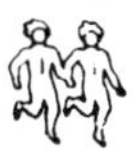 Gemini . . . . (May 21 — June 20)

 Cancer . . . . (June 21 — July 21)

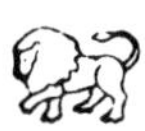 Leo . . . . (July 22 — August 21)

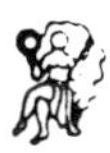 Virgo . . . . (August 22 — September 22)

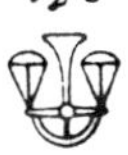 Libra . . . . (September 23 — October 23)

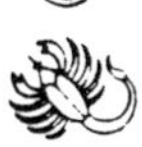 Scorpio . . . . . . (October 24 — November 21)

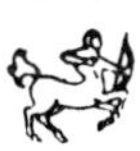 Sagittarius . . . (November 22 — December 21)

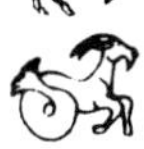 Capricorn . . . . . (December 22 — January 20)

Signs may be used as a part of a birthday party, or a star-gazing evening as constellations are located in the sky.

ACKNOWLEDGEMENTS

APPENDIX

CALENDARING THE YEAR

MANUAL ALPHABET

NUMERALS AND
SPECIAL SIGNS IF PATIENT IS DEAF

WISDOM GLEANED FROM ELDERS

ABOUT THE AUTHOR

ACKNOWLEDGEMENTS

One seldom embarks on a project such as this book without the aid of numerous individuals.

At the inception of the idea for a handbook Helen Spring was there to type from my tapes and notes, as I worked out my format, a decade ago.

Typist Catherine Wise assisted mightily in preparing first draft of the manuscript, even as she was experiencing remissions in her struggle with cancer.

To test the validity of this work I called upon Dr. Annette Logan, professor, Department of Therapeutic Recreation, York College of Pennsylvania, who read, and added helpful comments.

Early critical reader was Jean Heller, supervisor language arts Williamsport School District, Williamsport, Pennsylvania. Margaret Barnhart, retired editor and former colleague in the then editorial division of The Methodist Publishing House, Nashville, Tennessee, did a superb piece of work, editing my manuscript for publication.

A host of others served to critique, endorse, and affirm the rationale for such a book. Among these are:

Josephine Barley (Mrs. Marlin), personal care facility owner/manager.

Cindy Douglass, originator of Hospice, York, PA.

Cindy Erisman, O.T. with VNA, Alumnus of Elizabethtown College.

Judy Irwin, American Association University Women, former staff person local Area Agency on Aging.

Vera Long, Hospice Team Coordinator, VNA/Hospice, York, PA.

Carl Ford Peterson, CPE, York District Superintendent.

Linda Kay Peterson, LPN, Bethany Village Health-Care Facility, Mechanicsburg, PA.

Kimberly Pritchard, RMT-CMT, Alumnus Temple University contributed section on Music Therapy.

David Reed, NHA, Executive Director U.M. Continuing Care Service, Lewisburg, PA.

Patricia Runkle, Activities Director, Manor Care South Nursing and Rehabilitation Center provided list of resources for activities center.

Samuel Shultz, consultant, member Y.A.D., P.S.A.D., N.A.D.

Sally Arnold Suskin, R.N., art consultant.

Curtis and Eleanor Vinson, faithful volunteers, pictured throughout.

For permission from many to use random photos, illustrations, and quotations appearing in this book.

Gratitude to each abounds mightily. Thank you.

Laura R. Hess
Diaconal Minister (D.M.)

APPENDIX

CALENDARING SPECIAL EVENTS

Plan for the year of activity in a health care facility, or select out of the list below observances the senior citizen living in your home might enjoy, along with other family members or friends.

The following list is not official for the current year or month according to *Chase's Calendar of Annual Events*. These are offered to aid you in your planning.

JANUARY — Human Relations Month, March of Dimes Month, Eye Care Month, Oatmeal Month, Soup Month, Volunteer Blood Donor Month.

Special week or days: Official Man Watchers' Week, National Pizza Week, Chinese New Year (usually 2 weeks long). Martin Luther King Birthday, Hat Day, National Hugging Day, Popcorn Day, Superbowl Sunday, National Kazoo Day.

FEBRUARY — Heart Month, American History Month, Black History Month, Blah Buster Month.

Special days: Ground Hog Day, Norman Rockwell Birthday (1894), Babe Ruth Day (1895), Lincoln - Washington Celebrations, Valentine Day, Have a Heart Day, Race Relations Day, Mardi Gras and Shrove (Fat) Tuesday, Ash Wednesday, International Friendship Week.

MARCH — Nutrition Month, Peanut Month, Woman's History Month, Poetry Month, Red Cross Month.

Special days or weeks: National Pig Day, National Volunteers Week, Telephone Day (1st Message 1876), St. Patrick's Day, Earth Day — Spring Begins, Houdini Day (born 1874).

APRIL — Cancer Control Month, Holy Humor Month, Keep America Beautiful Month, National Occupational Therapy Month.

Special days or weeks: April Fools Day, National Garden Week, National Barbershop Quartette Day, Palm Sunday, Good Friday, Easter Sunday (moveable dates), National Library Week, National Intimate Apparel Week, Jewish Heritage Week.

MAY — Better Sleep Month, Better Hearing Month, Mental Health Month, Arthritis Month, Barbeque Month, Older American Month.

Special days or weeks: Mother Goose Day, Be Kind to Animals Week, National Family Week, National Nursing Home Week, National Tourism Week, National Nurses Day.

JUNE — Dairy Month, Adopt-a-Cat Month, Accordian Awareness Month, Zoo and Aquarium Month, Black Music Month. American Rivers.

Special days or weeks: Salvation Army Week, Donut Day, Teacher "Thank You" Week, Balloon Day - 1st Hot Air Flight (1789). National Flag Week, Smile Power Day, Father's Day (first celebrated 1910), Summer begins June 21 - have a picnic or barbecue.

JULY — Anti-boredom Month, Baked Bean Month, Hot Dog Month, Ice Cream Month, Hitch-hikers Month.

Special days: Independence Day, Canada Day.

AUGUST — National Catfish Month, National Water Quality Month.

Special day or week: Munchkins of Oz Convention.

SEPTEMBER — All-American Breakfast Month, National Cholesterol Education Month, National Courtesy Month.

Special days: Labor Day, Off-to-School Day.

OCTOBER — Consumer Information Month, National Adopt-a-Dog Month, National Clock Month, National Physical Therapy Month.

Special days: World-wide Communion Sunday (Protestant), Columbus Day, Canadian Thanksgiving Day, Day-light Saving Time Ends, Halloween.

NOVEMBER — Aviation History Month, National Alzheimers' Awareness Month, National Diabetes Month.

Special days: All Saints Day, Veterans Day, Election Day, Thanksgiving Day, National Bible Week.

DECEMBER — Advent, Hanukkah, Christmas, New Year's Eve, Watch Night.

MANUAL ALPHABET

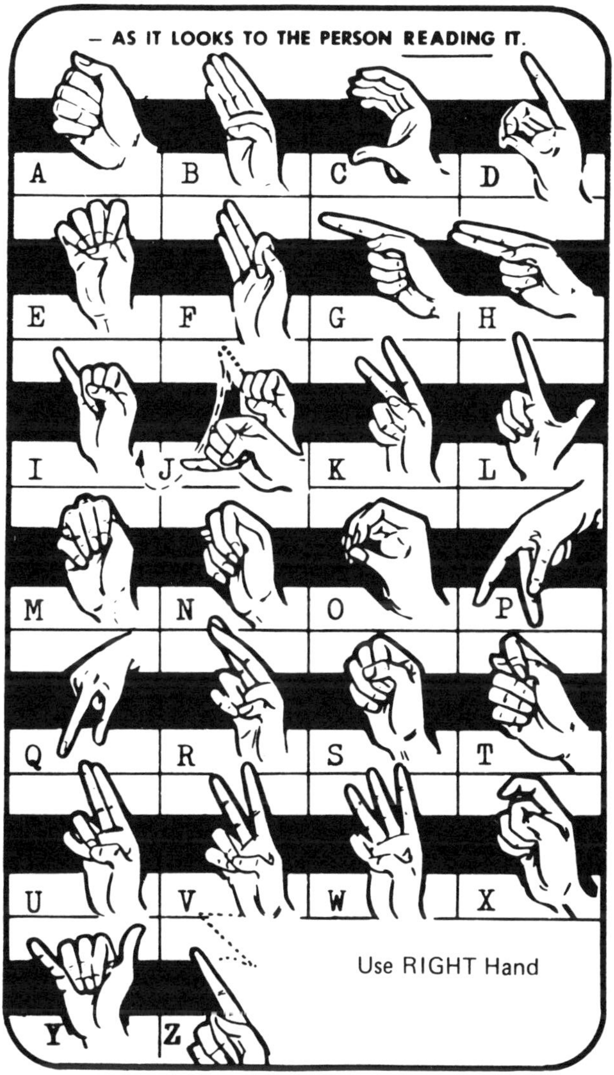

NUMERALS

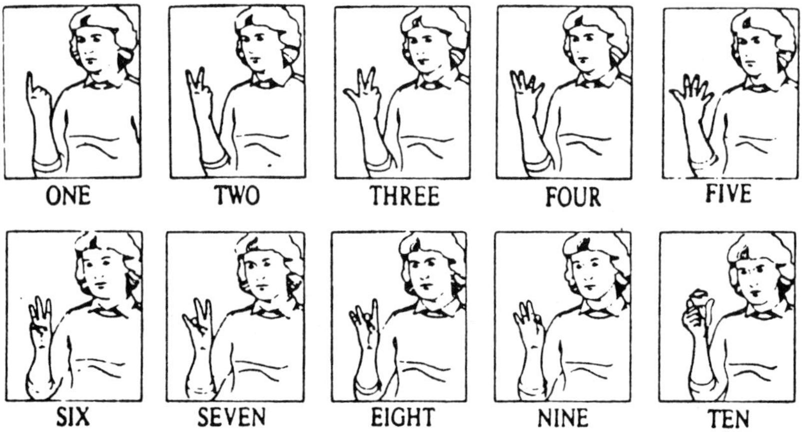

SPECIAL SIGNS IF PATIENT IS DEAF

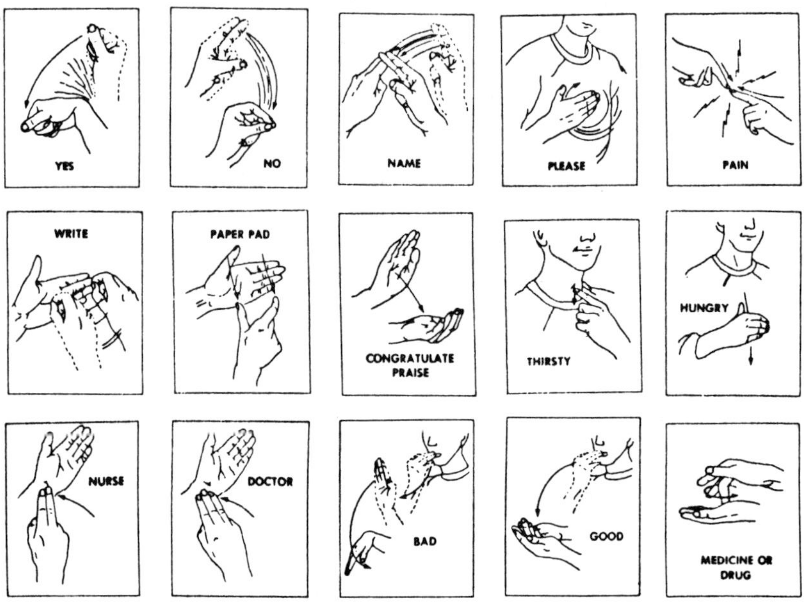

Courtesy
RN Magazine, June 1976
Illustrations by Shirley Baty

WISDOM I'VE GLEANED FROM WORKING WITH ELDERS

Samples to add to:

"I never read the paper until my morning chores are done. Better to read in the evening; then if I fall asleep work does not go wanting."

Elder neighbor, Mrs. Gertrude Arnold

"When you don't know what harbor your're sailing toward, no wind is a good one."

Tom Hopkins, grandfather

ABOUT THE AUTHOR

LAURA HESS, native of Williamsport, Pennsylvania, received her B.S. degree in Home Economics Education and English from Mansfield University, Mansfield, Pennsylvania and her M.A. degree from Scarritt College, Nashville, Tennessee, majoring in Social Group Work and Religious Education. As a certified director of Christian Education, she served churches in Florida, Detroit, Central New York, and Central Pennsylvania Conference of the United Methodist Church. Laura is also a diaconal minister in the United Methodist Church and serves as registrar for the Central Pennsylvania Conference Board of Diaconal Ministry.

She served as an editor of junior high curriculum materials for The Methodist Church supervising the development of a twelve-book curriculum . Writing articles and units of study for United Methodist periodicals and other publications for church school teachers continued through her years of employment as Christian education director.

Working closely with a deaf community she learned sign language, and assisted hard-of-hearing adults in developing a support group. Her ministry also included visitation in nursing home and hospital. In addition, Laura has taken courses in reality orientation and motivational therapy techniques.

In retirement she is a CONTACT worker, serves on a woman's health issues committee with American Association of University Women, York branch, and chairs May Fellowship Day celebrations for Church Women United of York County. Recently she served on the Church and Community Advisory Group for the development of a York United Methodist Home, a continuing and personal care facility in planning stage. She gardens, welcomes guests to her table, and shares her home with an occasional student and her Siamese cat.